T0259095

HANDBOOK FOR THE ASSESSMENT OF DRIVING CAPACITY

HANDBOOK FOR THE ASSESSMENT OF DRIVING CAPACITY

Edited by

Maria T. Schultheis, John DeLuca, and Douglas L. Chute

AMSTERDAM • BOSTON • HEIDELBERG • LONDON • NEW YORK • OXFORD
PARIS • SAN DIEGO • SAN FRANCISCO • SINGAPORE • SYDNEY • TOKYO
Academic Press is an imprint of Elsevier

Academic Press is an imprint of Elsevier
525 B Street, Suite 1900, San Diego, CA 92101-4495, USA
30 Corporate Drive, Suite 400, Burlington, MA 01803, USA
32 Jamestown Road, London NW1 7BY, UK
Radarweg 29, PO Box 211, 1000 AE Amsterdam, The Netherlands

First edition 2009

Notice
No responsibility is assumed by the publisher for any injury and/or damage to persons
or property as a matter of products liability, negligence or otherwise, or from any use
or operation of any methods, products, instructions or ideas contained in the material
herein. Because of rapid advances in the medical sciences, in particular, independent
verification of diagnoses and drug dosages should be made

Library of Congress Cataloging-in-Publication Data
A catalog record for this book is available from the Library of Congress

British Library Cataloguing in Publication Data
A catalogue record for this book is available from the British Library

ISBN: 978-0-12-631255-3

For information on all Academic Press publications
visit our website at books.elsevier.com

Typeset by Charon Tec Ltd., A Macmillan Company. (www.macmillansolutions.com)

Printed and bound in the USA
09 10   10 9 8 7 6 5 4 3 2 1

Working together to grow
libraries in developing countries

www.elsevier.com | www.bookaid.org | www.sabre.org

ELSEVIER   BOOK AID
International   Sabre Foundation

CONTENTS

3

DRIVING CONSULTATION AND INTERVENTION   35

ROSAMOND GIANUTSOS

PART II

TOPICS IN DRIVING RESEARCH   55

4

HUMAN FACTOR CONSIDERATIONS IN MOTOR VEHICLE COLLISIONS   59

PHILIP SCHATZ AND FRANK G. HILLARY

5

DRIVING AND TRAUMATIC BRAIN INJURY   71

C. ALAN HOPEWELL

6

DRIVING AND THE DEMENTIAS   95

GILLIAN K. FOX, ALAN HOPEWELL, EMILY ROSENMAN AND MARIA T. SCHULTHEIS

7

DRIVING AND STROKE   117

MARIA T. SCHULTHEIS AND CASSANDRA FLEKSHER

8

DRIVING AND OTHER NEUROLOGICAL AND PSYCHIATRIC DISORDERS   131

JESSICA H. KALMAR AND JOHN DELUCA

9

DRIVING, MEDICAL ILLNESS AND MEDICATIONS   159

THOMAS GALSKI, LORAN VOCATURO AND THOMAS M. GALSKI

10

DRIVING AND THE LAW   187

THOMAS GALSKI AND MARY ANNE McDONALD

11

FINAL THOUGHTS AND FUTURE DIRECTIONS   201

MARIA T. SCHULTHEIS

PREFACE

_____

In today's modern society there is little argument that the ability to drive an automobile is a critical component of an independent lifestyle. Indeed, an individual's reliance on personal transportation can have a direct impact on what they do for a living, how they socialize and for many how they define their autonomy. And while the reasons for driving may vary throughout an individual's lifetime, the importance of maintaining this privilege typically remains.

For an individual with a neurological compromise, these statements also hold true. However, these individuals are faced with potential impairments that may affect or limit and in some cases prohibit their ability to continue to remain on the road safely, yet the desire to maintain the driving privilege commonly remains. For clinicians working these individuals, the task of determining whether they are ready to return to driving can be daunting. This critical decision requires a balance of understanding the potential risk (to both the individual and others) and the impact to that individual's quality of life. Yet, it is important to recognize that for both clinician and patients, there is a common goal of allowing safe drivers to remain on the road.

HOW THIS BOOK CAME TO BE

This book is a basically the result of 12 years of learning from a great variety of people, including patients, colleagues, mentors, students and friends. Its existence is a result of many hours of observations, conversations and frustrations over what is a very scientifically complex and clinically challenging topic.

Early in my career, I had the opportunity to work in a community-based rehabilitation program for individuals who had sustained moderate to severe neurological compromise, most commonly from traumatic brain injury. During this early exposure, I learned first-hand the importance of maintaining the privilege to drive, by directly observing the incredible limitations in vocational and social opportunities and the emotional impact that resulted from the loss of this privilege. What was remarkable to me at that time was that there appeared to be a lack of consistency in how the determination of who could and could not drive was made. It was this question that fueled my initial interest in examining how clinicians address the task of evaluating and determining driving capacity.

Since this time, I have worked to expand my understanding of our current clinical approach to determining driving capacity. Through both research and clinical work I have observed both the strengths and weaknesses in our approach and have attempted to introduce new methods for meeting this important need. In addition to reviewing the clinical literature on driving, I have also turned to the transportation literature (and other fields) to expand my understanding the behavior of driving. In doing so, I have been surprised by the significant number of common issues addressed by these various areas of expertise that examine driving. Yet, I have been equally astounded by the lack of integration of this knowledge base into our clinical approaches.

Although the goal of understanding the very complex behavior of driving is a long term objective for me, along the way, it came to my attention that much of the knowledge from the research that has been conducted on driving with clinical populations is not readily available to clinicians who are charged with the responsibility of making this determination. It was this lack of resource that persuaded me to identify a mechanism for compiling this literature into a useful handbook for clinicians. Therefore, the goal of this book became to bring together and present the clinical understanding of driving assessment and rehabilitation.

HOW TO USE THIS BOOK

The material in the book is written for persons at a number of levels. One targeted audience is the group of clinicians who are faced with the task of evaluating driving capacity with little to no additional support. This can include individuals in private practices, in rural settings or in institutions that do not have an extended rehabilitation program with access to driver rehabilitation specialist. For these individuals, the book aims to provide an overview of the common aspects of driver assessment and a compilation of the clinical literature arranged by most common neurological disorders seen in rehabilitation. In addition the book provides some practical resources (e.g., state requirements, web based information) to aid these individuals in gathering information needed for making decisions and recommendations.

The book may also be helpful for those individuals who have clinical driving assessment expertise. For these individuals, the book provides a summary of the scientific studies and a quick reference for data related to important issues within specific neurological diagnoses. Additionally, the book underscores the importance of a multi-disciplinary, multi-level approach to driving and the value of integrating other disciplines (i.e., transportation literature). Clinicians conducting driving assessments may find this information useful for expanding their conceptualization of driving beyond the current clinical scope and potentially exploring new ways to enhance their current approach. Finally, this book is intended to introduce the area of clinical driving assessment and rehabilitation to the novice or student. The book is designed to be a relatively straight forward read that provides information about what has been studied and the vast amount of work that remains to be done in this field.

"THE ROAD TO SUCCESS IN STILL UNDER CONSTRUCTION"

Driving is one of the most complex behaviors that individuals perform because it requires the integration of a variety of physical, sensory, cognitive and emotional abilities. To add to the complexity, the behavior of driving is performed within an ever-changing environment and context that is often too difficult to predict or anticipate. That being said, it would be impossible for one book to cover all of the relevant aspects of driving. Subsequently, the current book is only one step in a large and ambitious undertaking that is being addressed by a variety of disciplines and expertise.

In general this book is designed to serves as a quick resource or reference that hopefully provides a glimpse into the clinical conceptualization of driving assessment. It is not all-inclusive but is meant to begin to compile our clinical knowledge in a manner that may help identify current weaknesses, as well as areas for future growth. It is my view that by first understanding the current state of the clinical driving literature, we can then begin to define where it should be going. The book is meant to encourage new thinking towards a multi- and trans-disciplinary approach to the clinical driving assessment. It is but one step in the long term objective of developing evidence-based tools to help inform clinical decision making about driving capacity.

ACKNOWLEDGEMENT

This book is dedicated to Al and Samantha, my two greatest sources of strength and perseverance—which was much need for the completion of this project! I also want to thank the numerous people in my life who have patiently tolerated my continued chatter about this topic, this includes many friends, students, colleagues and luckily for me one outstanding mentor (Dr. Douglas Chute) and one outstanding "professional guide" and friend (Dr. Joseph Ricker).

THE CLINICAL DRIVING ASSESSMENT

Driver rehabilitation can be defined as a component of rehabilitation medicine that specifically focuses on the evaluation and retraining of driving ability following a medical condition. To this end, a driver rehabilitation specialist is an individual who is capable of evaluating an individual's current driving ability, assesses driving potential and enables the person to return to safe, independent driving whenever possible.

While there is no clear date as to when driver rehabilitation began in the United States, in the 1950s and 1960s the growing number of rehabilitation hospitals led to an increase in professionals offering services of driver rehabilitation. To meet the growing need of these professionals, the Association of Driver Educators for the Disabled (ADED) was founded in 1977 primarily for the support of professionals working in the field of driver education and transportation equipment modification for persons with disabilities. The ADED founding members included a group of 30 individuals varying in background, including occupational therapists, driver educators, and equipment manufacturers. ADED became the first professional organization to advocate for professionals working in the field of driver assessment and driver retraining and helped to increase awareness and education about modification and adaptive equipment needs. However, one of ADED's most significant contribution to the field is its certification process, which was the first credentialing program for professionals in the field of driver rehabilitation.

Since its inception, driver rehabilitation has expanded in scope, but still faces challenges. In fact, one challenge faced by ADED and others in the field is the lack of federally mandated statutes and regulations, which results in significant variations of driver rehabilitation services and delivery. This need for the standardization has been identified by the National Highway Traffic Safety Administration (NHTSA, 2001) and work has been initiated toward this goal. In general, these organizations have strived to increase knowledge dissemination, provide guidelines and professional standards and increase public awareness about the importance of maintaining the privilege to drive following disabilities.

Despite its short history, the field of driver rehabilitation continues to grow and organizations such as ADED have helped to establish clinical guidelines and recommendations to this challenging component of rehabilitation medicine. It is the objective of "Part I: The Clinical Driver Assessment" to introduce the reader to the various components of driver rehabilitation services. This includes an overview of a driver evaluation (Chapter 1), which is a comprehensive assessment of the individual's ability and potential to become an independent driver and includes both on-road and off-road testing. The driver evaluation is the first phase in driver rehabilitation and lays the foundation for additional services, such as driver retraining and vehicle modification (Chapter 2).

It is important to note, that the information provided reflects practices within two established Driver Rehabilitation Programs, and as such may not be completely representative of the varying types of driver rehabilitation programs available today. Yet, these chapters describe what is typically considered the *gold standard* which includes evaluation and integration of medical history, visual functioning, physical and cognitive functioning and driving history.

It is also important to note, that although the contributing authors have extensive background and expertise in the field of driver rehabilitation, they represent only a small component of the largely diverse group that makes up driver rehabilitation. In general, the field of driver rehabilitation has attracted individuals from varying areas of expertise; however, to date driver rehabilitation has predominantly become a specialized field within occupational therapy. However, in practice it is not limited to occupation therapy and the task of assessing driving capacity can fall upon varying types of clinicians (e.g. physicians, psychologist). Furthermore, the task of determining driver capacity often requires input from various disciplines within rehabilitation medicine (e.g. physical therapist, neuropsychologists).

The first chapters serve to describe the elements of services provided within driver rehabilitation, including (1) driver evaluation, (2) driver retraining, and (3) vehicle modification. These chapters aim to introduce the reader to the terminology and the objectives and goals within these different types of clinical services.

PART

II

TOPICS IN DRIVING
RESEARCH

In the second component of this book our goal is to provide an overview of the driving research that has been conducted with clinical populations and to address some of the major topics in this area. In contrast to the first chapters, which described the clinical services that are commonly performed as part of a driver evaluation, this section aims to focus on the scientific studies and topics that have been raised and continue to be explored.

To commence this section, Chapter 4 begins with a discussion of factors that are known to contribute to motor vehicle collisions. Specifically this chapter presents basic descriptive and epidemiologic data characterizing motor vehicle collisions and the human and collision factors that influence their likelihood. In doing so, the chapter establishes a background for later chapters which will examine some of these factors from a clinical perspective.

This is followed by four chapters each covering specific diagnoses in relation to driving research. Because many of the early clinical studies examining driving after neurological compromise were focused on brain injury, Chapter 5 covers this literature by review-ing work examining driving after traumatic brain injury (TBI). This comprehensive review includes a discussion of the major issues in returning to driving after TBI, from both a medical and neuropsycho-logical perspective, as well as a discussion of concomitant issues that may arise secondary to TBI, such as pharmacological management. This is followed by Chapter 6, which covers a growing area in the clinical driving literature, driving and dementia. While this chapter focuses mainly on research related to dementia of the Alzheimer's type, a discussion of other types of dementia is also included. Specifically, the chapter reviews research that has examined assess-ment approaches with drivers with dementia and addresses relevant topics related to this older population, such as public policy issues (e.g., license renewal). In Chapter 7, the authors cover the diagno-sis that makes up the greatest percentage of the rehabilitation popu-lation, stroke or cerebral vascular accidents (CVA). This chapter highlights the key areas of research that have been covered with this population, including issues of right versus left hemisphere deficit, visual and visual perception issues and other influencing factors, such as aging and stroke. The final chapter in this segment is Chapter 8, which covers research examining driving among neurological dis-orders, specifically attention-deficit hyperactivity disorder (ADHD), multiple sclerosis (MS), epilepsy and includes a discussion of psy-chiatric disorders and driving. In contrast to many other clinical pop-ulations, work examining driving capacity among these individuals has recently been initiated and as such represents a growing research area in this field. The authors summarize the key studies and provide an overview of the salient issues related to these clinical groups.

The final segment includes three chapters designed to address relevant issues related to driving across clinical populations. In Chapter 9, the authors provide a comprehensive overview of the key issues related to medical and medication issues that can directly impact driving capacity. The authors first provide a discussion of medical issues that may not be directly related to a primary diag-nosis (such as brain injury or stroke) but may subsequently result in concomitant difficulties, such as cardiac or sleep disorders. The second part of the chapter provides clear descriptions of the different types of medications used to treat these disorders and discusses their potential side effects in relation to driving performance. This is followed by Chapter 10, which introduces some of the common legal issues that have been presented in the literature related to driving. This chapter discusses the important difference in laws and regulations that vary from state to state and discusses legal procedures in the evaluation of driving capacity, which apply to both medically and non-medically involved individuals.

The final chapter in this segment is designed to bring together what is presented in this book. To achieve this, this chapter first summarizes some of the common findings that can be drawn from the research conducted across the various clinical populations. These lessons learned are designed to provide the clinician with some practical recommendations that can be drawn from the literature and applied to everyday clinical practice. The second segment of this chapter then turns attention to what lies ahead and what challenges still remain in the arena of driving research.

In sum, the objective is to provide a comprehensive review of the existing work in driving and clinical populations. While, admittedly this is not all-inclusive, our objective was to provide solid introduction into what has been achieved.

CONTRIBUTORS

Numbers in parentheses indicate the pages on which the authors' contributions begin.

Agnes Agnelli (5) DMA Rehability, London, Ontario, Canada

Richard Nead (21) Kessler Institutes for Rehabilitation, West Orange, NJ

Rosamond Gianutsos (35) Cognitive Rehabilitation Services, Sunnyside, NY

Philip Schatz (59) Saint Joseph's University, Philadelphia, PA

Frank G. Hillary (59) Pennsylvania State University, University Park, PA

C. Alan Hopewell (71, 95) Clinical Neuropsychologist, Dallas, TX

Gillian K. Fox (95) Clinical Neuropsychologist, Hong Kong SAR, China

Emily, Roseman (95) Drexel University, Philadelphia, PA

Maria T. Schultheis (95, 117, 201) Drexel University, Philadelphia, PA

Cassandra Fleksher (117) Kessler Medical Rehabilitation & Research Corporation, West Orange, NJ

Jessica H. Kalmar (131) Yale School of Medicine, New Haven, CT

John DeLuca (131) Kessler Medical Rehabilitation Research and Education Corporation, West Orange, NJ

Thomas Galski (159, 187) Clinical Neuropsychologist, Colonia, NJ

Loran Vocaturo (159) Kessler Institutes for Rehabilitation Driver Rehabilitation Program, West Orange, NJ

Thomas M. Galski (159) The Cardiology Group, Medford, NJ

Mary Anne McDonald (187) Henry H. Kessler Foundation, West Orange, NJ

1

ON- AND OFF-ROAD

EVALUATIONS

AGNES AGNELLI

The assessment of one's ability to drive after a physical or cognitive insult is a challenging task on a variety of levels. Legally, it is typically a physician's obligation to report a change in medical status to the licensing bureau of the province/state. Physicians are often in the precarious situation of determining whether the specific insult has impacted the individual's ability to drive. However, they lack the specific assessment tools and skills to adequately determine this with certainty in their office/clinics. Subsequently, many physicians will prescribe a driving evaluation to aid in their determination of driving capacity following physical or cognitive compromise.

Today driver evaluations can be conducted by independently practicing driver specialist, as well as within the context of specialized driver assessment programs. The latter are typically associated with larger physical medicine and rehabilitation institutions. Although there remains considerable variability in what constitutes a driver evaluation, there is some level of consensus that both on road (e.g., behind-the-wheel evaluations) and off road (e.g., perceptual testing) are important elements. The aim of this chapter is to present these key elements by describing a current clinical driver assessment program that aims to objectively and systematically determine an individual's ability to drive following a physical and/or cognitive insult.

BACKGROUND

Galski et al. (1990) found that results of in-clinic testing (perceptual and neuropsychological tests) did not correlate with evaluating the skills and abilities required for safe driving. They suggest that the pre-driver evaluation (in-clinic testing) should not be used as a predictor of driving performance, but rather a screening tool to identify those clients who would be unsafe behind the wheel. In their 1998 review, Fox et al. recommend the use of a dual-control vehicle during behind-the-wheel evaluations. They suggested that both testing and scoring procedures need to be standardized if on-road assessment is to have a high validity. They noted that specifying objective criteria for adequate driving performance could lead to objective scoring of performance during the on-road evaluation. The authors also commented on closed-course assessments. They indicated that these assessments evaluate basic car maneuvering skills, including maintaining the car in a straight course, ability to drive through cones and braking. However, they cautioned that the closed-course assessment does not evaluate the ability of the individual to interpret and react with other drivers; lacks ecological validity; and while it may be useful to determine whether a client meets the minimum standards of competence, it does not test the skill for driving in complex situations.

Katz et al. (1990) concluded in their study that the brain-damaged patients who passed a comprehensive driving assessment were as fit to drive as their matched controls. The comprehensive driving assessment consisted of:

- A medical assessment (including history and physical examinations; vision; lack of seizure disorder; evaluation of fatigue, ability to read and understand instructions; lack of disordering mood).
- Evaluation by driving specialist which included visual testing, reaction time assessment, driving simulation and behind-the-wheel evaluation.
- A psychological evaluation by a neuropsychologist, including an extended mental status exam in conjunction with a neuropsychological test battery.

In reviewing the above literature, it is clear that the findings supports both in-clinic and behind-the-wheel assessment in determining an individual's ability to drive. As such, it is not surprising that in clinical practice the most common approach to evaluating driving capacity following many medical conditions is through a comprehensive driving evaluation. The key elements to a comprehensive driving evaluation have been defined as: (1) a pre-driving evaluation, (2) an in-clinic or off-road assessment, and (3) a behind-the-wheel or on-road assessment. Although federal requirements vary from state-to-state in the United States and currently there is a lack of standardization, some organizations, such as ADED, have supported the recommendation for a comprehensive driving evaluation and have provided recommendations and guidelines for therapist conducting these evaluations. The remainder of this chapter will attempt to describe the various elements of this complex evaluation.

THE COMPREHENSIVE DRIVING EVALUATION

PRE-DRIVING EVALUATION

The evaluator who has the task of determining fitness to drive typically has limited time and information available to him/her at the time of the assessment. Therefore, collection of pertinent medical information prior to the assessment is critical in order to maximize the effectiveness of the assessment. Furthermore, individuals who undergo a driving evaluation often must pay for this service out-of-pocket and subsequently, cost-containment for the evaluation must be weighed against having the ideal amount of information to make a determination of the client's ability to drive. Offering a financially viable assessment requires the evaluation to be efficient, the evaluator to be knowledgeable regarding driving evaluations and the population whom they are assessing, and the evaluator to have adequate resources available to him/her to execute the assessment in a timely and cost-effective manner.

While, there are variety of sources of information that may assist the therapist in preparing for the driver evaluation, Table 1.1 summarizes key areas that should be examined/considered prior to the evaluation. Information from these areas can assist the evaluator to focus on predetermined identified areas of potential concern during both the in-clinic and in-car evaluation.

TABLE 1.1   Considerations Prior to Evaluation.

Area	Considerations
Vision	Request that the client provide an updated optometrist report that clearly indicates the client's vision meets the provincial/state standards.
Diagnosis	Obtain consent from the client to contact the treating physician regarding diagnosis that led to necessity of a Driving Evaluation (this may or may not be necessary depending on the evaluator's knowledge and experience in dealing with the particular diagnosis). See Appendix A.
Medical history	Prior to the evaluation, send questionnaire to the client soliciting information that may impact on the client's ability to drive (this may not be the reason for the evaluation) that is, diabetic with parasthesia who had a stroke (the latter being the reason for the evaluation, but the parasthesia may affect ability to drive). See Appendix B.
Driving history	Contact the provincial/state licensing authority to determine status. Status Obtain temporary driver's licence for on-the-road assessment. Often there is time required in order to obtain a temporary driver's licence. Each province/state will have its own system for obtaining this information.

IN-CLINIC/OFF-ROAD EVALUATION

The in-clinic evaluation provides the assessor with the necessary information to determine basic safety for progression to the behind-the-wheel/on-road assessment. Further, it provides cognitive and physical information to alert the evaluator to potential problem areas during the behind-the-wheel assessment. Rarely will it absolutely determine an individual's ability to safely drive.

To date, an assessment or battery of tests has not been developed which can conclusively determine an individual's ability to drive without the practical behind-the-wheel assessment. In extreme cases, where it is clear that the client does not exhibit the basic skills to drive, this is usually indicative of poor screening of the referral prior to the in-clinic evaluation. An example of this would be an individual who has sustained a stroke and has a left visual neglect. Such a referral would be considered premature and the in-clinic evaluation would help to identify this. As a result succession to the behind-the-wheel assessment would not occur.

As with the pre-evaluation there are a variety of areas that can be examined during the in-clinic. Table 1.2 summarizes key areas which should be assessed. The amount of time spent in each area will depend on the diagnosis of the client

TABLE 1.2   Areas of Assessment During In-Clinic/Off-Road Evaluation.

Area	Considerations
History taking	<ul><li>Current and past-medical history</li><li>Medications</li><li>Driving history (including years of experience, involvement in motor vehicle accidents, training, usual driving environment, vehicle type).</li></ul>
Physical assessment	<ul><li>Range of motion in upper and lower extremity</li><li>Muscle tone</li><li>Strength and endurance</li><li>Coordination and balance</li><li>Sensation and proprioception</li><li>Mobility</li><li>Vision (acuity, peripheral, depth perception).</li></ul>
Cognitive assessment	<ul><li>Memory</li><li>Attention (selective, divided and sustained)</li><li>Information processing speed</li><li>Problem solving and multi-tasking</li><li>Judgment</li><li>Visual perception</li><li>Ability to follow directions</li><li>Behavior (e.g. impulsivity, lack of awareness).</li></ul>
Driving knowledge	<ul><li>Road sign recognition</li><li>Rules of the road.</li></ul>

which prompted the driving evaluation in the first place. The assessor should, at minimum, do a screen of all areas to ensure that nothing is overlooked. The extent and thoroughness each area should be assessed is typically at the discretion of the evaluator. In order to maintain cost-effectiveness and still allow sufficient time to gather all necessary information, 1.5 hours of in-clinic assessment time should be allocated. This will be sufficient time in the majority of cases. It may be excess in situations where there are no cognitive concerns; however, it permits the evaluator the ability to assess cognition if alerted to a potential problem in this area (which may not have been flagged prior to the assessment).

BEHIND-THE-WHEEL/ON-ROAD ASSESSMENT

Implementing a comprehensive driving evaluation requires both in-clinic/off-road and behind-the-wheel/on-road assessments. Deciding when to conduct the latter of these, either same day as in-clinic or on another day, can be influenced by various factors. In many cases, given the time limitations to both therapist and clients, the behind-the-wheel evaluation is typically scheduled on the same day of the in-clinic. However, there are both negative and positive aspects to this approach.

Pros for evaluating on the same day

- Evaluator has the results of the in-clinic evaluation at hand and can more efficiently link this to the on-road assessment (no need to review the in-clinic results prior to the on-road assessment).
- Client has the results of the assessment in a timely manner, without delay.
- Client does not have to make two trips to the evaluation center.
- Avoids scheduling difficulties on two different days.

Cons to evaluating on the same day

- In-clinic evaluation may indicate that on-road assessment is not appropriate – evaluator time already booked for the on-the-road assessment.
- Information that was not available prior to assessment can be further investigated, if necessary.
- Fatiguing process for the client to complete all in one day.

It is this author's assertion that same-day in-clinic and on-road assessment is a more practical situation. Appropriate screening of referrals, coupled with a comprehensive pre-evaluation and the education of referring sources, should minimize inappropriate referrals which may result in no behind-the-wheel evaluation. In those instances where more information is required after a comprehensive pre-evaluation and in-clinic, the behind-the-wheel assessment can be rescheduled for another day. This occurs so rarely that it does not justify making the assessment over 2 days a norm. Finally, the effect of fatigue on driving performance is important for the evaluator to observe and may impact on the evaluator's recommendations.

For the clients who lack insight into their driving potential (or lack thereof), the assessment often gives them the concrete proof that they do not possess the necessary skills to drive. Subsequently, providing the in-clinic and behind-the-wheel consecutively, may assist in educating and increasing the awareness of the client. Furthermore, reaching this conclusion in a timely manner may alleviate the burden of family members, who are often left with the task of explaining and convincing their loved one that they do not possess the ability to drive.

The recommended guidelines for a behind-the-wheel evaluation involves two therapists, an occupational therapist and certified driving instructor, and the client in a dual-control vehicle. The occupational therapist will typically discuss potential areas of concern with the driving instructor prior to initiation of the in-car evaluation. One hour for the in-car evaluation should be permitted. The assessment typically occurs during daylight hours.

Typically, driving starts in a quieter, residential area where there are few distractions and the demands are less. If the client is able to demonstrate good driving skills in this area, progression to more complex driving situations is initiated (see below). The behind-the-wheel evaluation, should include at minimum driving conditions which will allow observation of performance at right and left turns, stops (stop sign, traffic light, entering traffic area, four-way stop intersections), the ability to navigate and/or locate street addresses and the ability to drive in varying environments (residential, commercial, highway). The in-car assessment should also include:

- Orientation to the vehicle
  Advise client of specific controls (i.e., gear shift, rear/side mirrors, lights, windshield wipers).

- Overview of process
  Instructor should try and put client at ease. Reassure client that the process will look at client's ability to drive in normal driving situations. Advise client that he/she should drive as they normally drive. Typical introduction could be:

We will spend the next 30 minutes with you driving. I will give you specific instructions as to what I would like you to do, always giving you ample time to complete the request. Drive as you normally drive and always remember to keep safety first. I will not try and trick you or make you do something that is not safe. I will observe how you handle the vehicle, obey the rules of the road, and interact with the traffic. I have a brake on my side of the vehicle, and will use it if I feel it is necessary to stay safe. During the first 30 minutes, my job is to give you directions as to where to go. I will not point out any errors or give you tips on improving your performance. After this time, we will stop and I will point out any concerns I may have, and may ask you to do some things to improve your driving. We will drive for an additional 10–15 minutes, making our way back to the centre. We will then review your overall driving performance with any recommendations at that time. Do you have any questions?

- Presentation of complex driving situations, such as:

1. Lane changes in four lane city streets (i.e., "When it's safe to do so, make a lane change to the left").
2. Right-hand turn at an intersection (i.e., "At the next set of lights, make a right-hand turn").
3. Left-hand turn at a side street (i.e., "Make a left-hand turn at the next available street").
4. Left-hand turn at an intersection (i.e., "Turn left at the next set of lights").
5. Client to make a decision regarding road sign without cuing (i.e., client proceeding toward a "Do Not Enter Sign", AND/OR client proceeding straight and to a T-intersection where there is a one-way street, instructor advises "Continue, obeying the signs").
6. Introduce conversation into the evaluation to determine how client is able to maintain concentration with this distraction.
7. Incorporate a delay from delivery of an instruction and client executing the instruction (i.e., client progressing straight on a road and no opportunity to make a right-/left-hand turn for several blocks. Instructor advises "Make a left-hand turn at the next available light").
8. If client is familiar with the city, ask him/her to return the vehicle to the assessment center.

- *Recording of observed driving performance*
  Performance on the behind-the-wheel evaluation can be recorded through the use of a behind-the-wheel performance checklist. While, this is not a requirement and currently there is no standardized checklist available, many driving evaluators have developed individual checklists that are used to incorporate their observations during the behind-the-wheel evaluation (refer to Appendix C). Ideally, performance observations are recorded during driving typically by the second evaluator; however, in many cases, where only one evaluator is available, the checklist is completed immediately following the behind-the-wheel. The use of a performance checklist can assist therapist in recording their observations, but can also provide a mechanism for objectifying and quantifying their evaluation of the client's driving performance. Additionally, the performance ratings of the client during the behind-the-wheel can help identify specific areas of difficulties the individual may be experiencing.

During the behind-the-wheel evaluation, the therapist may have the opportunity to observe how findings from the in-clinic/off-road assessment impact the individual's ability to drive an automobile. Although, empirical data for the relationship between in-clinic measures and specific driving behaviors do not exist,

Table 1.3 provides some examples of how some in-clinic findings may affect on-the-road performance.

It is critical for the driving instructor and/or the occupational therapist to determine what client driving characteristics are due to the medical condition that brought them to the evaluation, and what is due to driving experience/habit. For example, an inexperienced driver with a mild brain injury should not be expected to perform better than an inexperienced driver without a brain injury. The expertise of both the evaluator and the driving instructor is critical in making this important distinction. An inexperienced driver may be hesitant in certain driving maneuvers (e.g., lane changes, left-hand turns, require more intense concentration). This should not necessarily be attributed to the effects of the cognitive impairment or given greater weight to overall driving performance. The benchmark for succeeding in the driving evaluation should match the licensing authority's criteria. The client should not be held to a higher standard than that imposed on them by the licensing body. Similarly, an older driver with a brain injury may never have been in the habit of checking blind spots. While the evaluation cannot support this behavior, it should not be attributed to the medical condition initiating the need for a driving evaluation. Rather, instruction to the client of the need to check his/her blind spot should be provided. The client's ability to incorporate this into his/her driving repertoire is far more indicative of

TABLE 1.3   In-Clinic/Off-Road Findings and Their Impact on Behind-the-Wheel Performance.

Deficit	Effect on-road performance
Attention/Concentration	• Easily detracted • Difficulty with multi-tasking • Not recognizing potential hazards • Poor lane positioning.
Information processing	• Slow reaction time to stimuli • Slow driving • Does not take in the whole scene • Makes correct decision too late • Stops at the last minute.
Judgment	• Risk-taking behavior • Poor problem solving • Poor analysis of situation with poor solution.
Insight	• Poor error recognition • Unable to identify reason for being there • Poor use of recommended strategies • No responsibility – blames others for situation.
Impulsivity	• Poor decision-making • Fast response – no problem solving • Limited observation of whole scene.

the client's ability, or potential ability to drive, than the actual omission of this driving habit.

MAKING THE DECISION

It is rare that upon completion of the in-clinic and on-the-road assessment that the client's ability to drive is a definitive YES or NO. The majority fall into the questionable category, typically leaving the responsibility of making the correct decision to the clinician and the driving instructor.

As noted earlier, one of the most challenging aspects of making this decision, is being able to separate what is habitual driving behavior and what behaviors are a result of impairment (such as poor visual processing speed). Some examples, of these different behaviors are provided in Table 1.4.

If the deficit areas are noted as occurring primarily in the "habitual" area, with good performance in the "impairment" area, this may be indicative of poor driving habits or inexperience. Opportunity to correct identified deficits should be incorporated into the driving evaluation. If there are numerous deficits identified in the "impairment" area, this may be indicative of cognitive/perceptual deficits and will require further intervention. If the client does not demonstrate the ability to integrate new information into learning or has poor insight into the deficits, the benefit of training should be considered.

To further assist in determining the individual's capacity to drive, the therapist's experience in conducting on-road evaluations can incorporated. Again, while little empirical evidence exist for this, clinical expertise cannot be ignored in the decision-making process. As such, there are a number of typically

TABLE 1.4   Examples of Driving Behavior Errors Resulting from Habitual Driving or Impaired Driving.

Habitual	Impairment
Rolling beyond stop sign	Moving in/out of traffic inappropriately
Stopping before a line	Straddling lanes
Poor blind spot check	Late braking when distracted
Poor mirror use	Leaving unsafe gap in traffic when attempting to make lane change
No checking of cross-traffic	Unawareness of traffic flow/pedestrian movement
Poor road sign recognition	Inconsistent signal use
Disregarding yellow light	Poor acknowledgment of stop signs/lights
Disobeying speed	Inconsistent wide/sharp turns, depending on activity distractions occurring at time
Consistent wide/sharp turns	Inability to react appropriately to immediate situation

impaired on-road behaviors which appear to be more frequently exhibit by cognitively impaired (regardless of originating source) clients, these can include:

- hesitating/stopping at green lights;
- poor positioning of vehicle in relation to road/other cars;
- consistently driving below the speed limit;
- impulsivity/risk-taking behaviors;
- unsafe left turns (may be related to impulsivity or poor judgment);
- changing lanes without awareness of surrounding vehicles:
- getting lost;
- poor road sign recognition;
- reduced awareness of other vehicles on the road;
- poor judgment.

RECOMMENDATIONS TO CLIENT

Finally, upon integrating all of the information gathered from the pre-evaluation, the in-clinic/off-road assessment and the behind-the-wheel/on-road assessment, a final recommendation is made to the client about their driving status. Typically, this recommendation will fall under one of the following categories:

1. *Resume driving*: Demonstrates good driving ability – no concerns.

2. *Requires training*: Client demonstrated some deficits in general driving performance. Poor integration of ability and implementation of rules of the road. Does demonstrate insight and the potential to learn strategies to improve driving ability OR requires practice with modified vehicle if problems are physical. While a definitive number of lessons cannot be anticipated, the amount of training depends on deficit area and client's learning ability. It is better to modestly over-estimate the number of lessons and not use all recommended lessons, particularly in the case of third party funding. Communication between the evaluator and driving instructor is important to determine when a re-evaluation should occur. A re-evaluation by the driving center may be necessary before licensing authority will consider re-issue of licence. As there will be an additional cost for the re-evaluation, it should be completed when the client has mastered the skills identified as problem areas during the initial evaluation to avoid incurring unnecessary costs.

3. *Further rehabilitation*: Client demonstrates the basic skill to become a safe driver; however, not yet ready to initiate driver training. In this situation, the referral source should be educated regarding appropriate timing for re-testing. In this situation, the client has demonstrated the ability to integrate new information into practice, but is not ready to do so in driver training.

4. *Disqualification*: The client does not demonstrate the required skills for driving, and does not demonstrate the ability to learn the necessary skills required for driving (inability to learn new information).

While some evaluators may make it their practice to err on the side of caution limiting their liability in making a wrong or premature decision, the majority of the recommendations fall under the "resume driving" or "requires training" category. In some situations, particularly in a progressive illness (early dementia, multiple sclerosis), the client may have demonstrated the ability to drive safely, but the rate of acceleration of the disease process is not known. In this case, the evaluator should highlight to the client and referral source that the need for a re-evaluation will be necessary as disease-related symptoms progress. This alleviates responsibility of the evaluator from liability in the case of progression of the disease and impact on safe driving ability.

REFERENCES

Fox, G., Bowden, S. C., & Smith, D. M. (1998). On-road assessment of driving competence after brain impairment: Review of current practice and recommendations for standardized examination. *Arch. Phys. Med. Rehabil.*, *79*(10), 1288–1296.

Galski, T., Ehle, H. T., & Bruno, R. L. (1990). An assessment of measures to predict the outcome of driving evaluations in patients with cerebral damage. *Am. J. Occup. Ther.*, *44*(8), 709–713. ISSN: 0272-9490.

Katz, R. T., Golden, R. S., Butter, J., Tepper, D., Rothke, S., Holmes, J., & Sahgal, V. (1990). Driving safety after brain damage: Follow-up of twenty-two patients with matched controls. *Arch. Phys. Med. Rehabil.*, *71*(2), 133–137. ISSN: 0003-9993.

APPENDIX A
PRE-EVALUATION QUESTIONNAIRE

1. Describe the medical problems for which this driving assessment is needed.

2. List any other medical conditions that you have now.

3. List all of the medications that you are taking presently (add another sheet if you need to):

Name of drug	Dose	How often?	How long have you taken it?
Example: Naproxen	375 mg	Twice daily	2 months
_____	_____	_____	_____
_____	_____	_____	_____

4. Are you presently receiving rehabilitation services such as occasional therapy or physiotherapy?

   ☐ Yes   ☐ No   If yes, list these services and where you are receiving them.

5. Are you driving now?

   ☐ Yes   ☐ What type of vehicle?
   ☐ No   ☐ When did you stop driving? Why?

6. Do you have concerns about your ability to drive? Please specify.

7. Do you have a valid driver's licence?   ☐ Yes ☐ No
   What is your licence number? _____   Exp. Date: _____
   If no, why?

8. Do you use any adaptive equipment such as a cane, wheelchair, scooter? Please specify.

9. Please include a copy of a recent (within last 3 months) eye examination completed by an optometrist.

APPENDIX B
REQUEST FOR REFERRAL INFORMATION

Dear Dr. _____ :

Your patient, _____, has been referred for an Occupational Therapy Driving Evaluation. As part of the evaluation, I require you to complete the following form to ensure that from a medical point of view, there are no contraindications for the patient to participate in this assessment. It will also provide me with necessary information to complete a thorough assessment. I must receive this back before an appointment can be booked with the patient.

Name of patient: _____ Date of birth:_____

Medical Diagnosis Necessitating Driving Evaluation:_____

Prognosis: This patient's condition is likely to (please check):

improve_____   deteriorate_____   remain stable

List other medical conditions, medications, allergies, emotional state, etc., that may affect this patient's ability to drive:_____
_____
_____

In your opinion, can this patient participate in an Occupational Therapy Driving Evaluation?   Yes_____   No_____

If no, please indicate rationale for same and the time frame when this may be able to occur._____

Please include any other information that may assist in this evaluation:
_____
_____
_____

Physician's Name (please print)   Address
_____   _____
_____   _____

                                             _____
Signature   Date

Thank you for your time in completing this questionnaire. Please include any reports/documentation that may be pertinent. A copy of the report will be forwarded to you upon its completion.

APPENDIX C
BEHIND-THE-WHEEL ASSESSMENT

Date: _____   Area: _____   Road/Weather:_____

Start: _____   Finish:_____   Modifications: _____

Key: **(S) = Satisfactory**   **(M) = Marginal**   **(U) = Unsatisfactory**

Skill	S	M	U	Comments
• Uses mirrors appropriately				
• Checks blind spot when appropriate				
• Checks left/right at intersection				
Communication				
• Appropriate use of turn signals				
• Uses horn as appropriate				
• Reads and obeys road signs				
Speed adjustment				
• Adjusts according to driving conditions				
• Adjusts according to road situation (i.e., construction, curves)				
• Excessively slow driving				
• Excessive acceleration				
• Adjusts for passing, crossing/turning at an intersection				
Vehicle positioning				
• Maintains safe gap in traffic				
• Yields space to other drivers when appropriate				

Selects correct lane before/during/ after turn				
Positions vehicle out of other drivers' blind spots				
Vehicle positioning				
• Appropriate merging into traffic				
• Vehicle maintained in appropriate				
• Turns completed without excessively sharp or wide turns				
Tactical performance				
• Responds appropriately to traffic emergencies				
• Responds appropriately to changing environment (i.e., city, □ highways, inclement weather)				
• Searches driving environment				
Behavior				
• Responds to feedback				
• Does not display aggressiveness				
• Does not display impulsiveness				
• Displays insight into driving habits/constructive criticism				
• Does not display risk-taking behavior				

Client: _____

Driver's licence: _____

Examiner: _____

2

DRIVER RETRAINING AND ADAPTIVE EQUIPMENT

RICHARD NEAD

Operation of a motor vehicle is a complex task requiring the interaction of several cognitive, sensory, and physical systems. Coupled with the ever changing driving environment providing countless obstacles and hazards, it is no wonder that at times it can overwhelm even the best of vehicle operators. A person with a disability may find the odds much greater in becoming an efficient driver. Depending on the type of disability and its severity, these individuals may be precluded from the independence that personal transportation can provide in one's life.

Granting this opportunity to persons with disabilities is commonly the charge of Driver Rehabilitation Programs (DRP) and the Driver Rehabilitation Specialists (DRS). The effective provision of these services can enhance an individual's capacity to gain independence through mobility. Although formidable, many obstacles can be overcome through proper evaluation and training. Fortunately, advances in the field of driver rehabilitation and in mobility technology have brought the potential for driving to many, who just a few short years ago would have had few opportunities regarding personal transportation. Evaluation and training can be obtained through a comprehensive DRP, administered by individuals with expertise in this field, such as Certified Driver Rehabilitation Specialists (CDRS). These individuals are persons with this knowledge and expertise who have passed a certification examination and are required to remain abreast of current trends in the field in order to maintain their credentials.

In order to successfully address the driving needs of individuals with disabilities, driver specialists must be capable of taking a skill or task, and breaking it down into simple, understandable components. They must also be capable of taking a raw talent and guiding this talent in becoming an accomplished performer.

In doing so, the driver specialist affords the opportunity for individuals with disabilities to develop a solid foundation from which they can strive to develop intermediate and advanced skills through further instruction and repetitions in the task. The aim of the chapter is to provide an overview of the current approach to providing additional instruction and training as part of reintegrating individuals with disabilities back into the driving community.

DRIVER REMEDIATION/TRAINING

For most individuals, driver remediation/training typically follows successful completion of the referral, interview, and pre-driver evaluations. The on-road or behind-the-wheel (BTW) assessment has been conducted, conferences between professionals have been completed, and the results have been discussed with the individual. Driver remediation is often recommended when findings during the BTW evaluation indicate the need for further intervention.

Prior to training it is important that several factors be determined during the evaluation. This information will assist in developing a productive training format. For example, the determination of driver experience. In the case of experienced drivers, it would be necessary to determine areas of deficiency that require remediating. By contrast, in the case of the new or newer operators, it would be necessary to determining the capacities for learning new tasks and improvement through repetition. This information can help the driver specialist in determining what skills need to be addressed, in what type driving environment they should be attempted, and the intensity in which repetition should be planned.

In most cases vehicle choice, adaptations, and modifications have also been determined during the evaluation performance. Training will solidify these choices or indicate the need to modify some or all of these initial recommendations. It is also common to have a projected number of sessions that will be required to reach the training goals. Length of sessions may vary particularly if difficulties with endurance (both physical and mental) are observed. The rate of progressions through the program is an individual factor which is governed by several issues, including:

- Is the operator experienced or are they new or newer to the driving task.
- How involved is the disability being dealt with and what is the degree of adversity for the individual.
- How is the individual learning to live with the disability and how well are they compensating.
- How well can the individual adapt and compensate for deficiencies in performance.
- How quickly and efficiently can the individual respond to new information and technologies.

In many instances how the specialist determines this information and deploys a corrective strategy will affect the ability and rate of an individual's success.

Finally, regardless of it being a training or remediation session, there is typically a continuous state of evaluating an individual's performance. This overall assessment of behaviors and skills can be helpful in determining what strategies are best employed in performance enhancement. This ongoing review process both separate and apart of instruction is imperative in providing optimal opportunity for the individual's success.

DRIVER REMEDIATION AND IMPROVED PERFORMANCE PROGRAM (DRIPP)

The DRIPP program was designed to help driver specialist teach/coach fundamental driving skills, compensating techniques, and improvement strategies. Although, federal regulations do not exist regarding delivery of driver retraining services, several organizations (e.g., ADED) have encouraged structure and standardization to help improve the overall efficacy of driver remediation/training. The DRIPP program is an example of this attempt to clearly define recommended procedures.

Preparation is a critical component of a successful training session. Reviewing an individual's evaluation results and any previous training sessions can provide critical information for determining the focus of the training session. It also allows the driver specialist to set goals for the daily session and realize if the pathways chosen are on target to meet them. Review and revision of goals may need to be visited after each session depending on that individual's progress in the program.

As specialists the goal is to develop a confident/competent level of performance in all individuals. This will include the teaching and repeating of fundamental and defensive driving skills to both experienced and inexperienced operators. This, as noted previously, can demand different training objectives and techniques. For example, after teaching a new driver the fundamentals of vehicle operation you may begin to introduce basic learning techniques. Whereas with an experienced driver, you may be revisiting fundamental skills so they can be performed with the use of hand-controls. As both develop and redevelop confidence in their performance, it will be necessary to give adequate repetition to allow progress to more advanced training sequences, once the carryover is complete. Carryover will need to be displayed on a consistent basis in multiple traffic scenarios. Various traffic densities should be explored exposing the student to several situations in which they must display their developed skills.

FUNDAMENTAL SKILLS

Preparation to Drive

The first of the fundamental skills to be taught or observed are the preparation to driver sequences. The first component, evaluated as the individual enters the vehicle, requires observation of their transfer efficiency. Difficulties with transfer into vehicle may be alleviated through the use of adaptive devices, training, and repetition. Normally this situation is governed by disability limitations and often compensating techniques can be taught to alleviate any difficulties. Once in the vehicle, it is necessary for the operators to independently achieve a safe driving position. The seat should first be adjusted, followed by seat belt, and mirror adjustment. If not completed in this order, one will undo the other, and create a hardship both prior to and being underway.

Second, the procedure to start the car and shift the car should be explained and several repetitions provided. Once the client becomes familiar with these sequences they should require very little of your training time. It is important to recall that for experienced operators, the "Driver Training" car will, at first, be unfamiliar to them. Explanation of the various operational details in clear, concise terms is important during this introduction to the vehicle. It is also helpful at this stage, to demonstrate the instructor's dual control system and clarify how they work. Clarification of the devices and the overall expectation can help to reassure safety at this early stage.

Movement

Initial movements of the vehicle will include the teaching of the skills of braking, accelerating, driving straight, and making basic left and right turns. Basic scanning instruction focused on looking up and out in front of the car versus looking down should be stressed. Clients with vision deficiencies should be made aware of this and in this low impact setting, cued to check areas of weakness often. Also early on, bringing in the use of the inside rearview and outside side view mirrors is important. For example, for experienced drivers, it should be noted if this is a part of their scanning ritual. In the case of new drivers, training individuals to check the rearview mirror whenever slowing or stopping can be introduced at this stage.

Introduction of basic defensive driving approaches can be included at varying points of driver training. For example, introducing the search/scan, identify, predict, decide and execute functions (SIPDE) of the defensive driving approach during low density or impact driving scenarios. In these less demanding situations a demonstration of this process can be provided and then have the individual use "commentary driving" principles in exhibiting their capacities. "Commentary driving" is a technique used when the individual tells you what it is they are seeing as they move through the driving environment. It is very useful in depicting how one is dividing their attentions while operating the motor vehicle.

The development and use of a driver curriculum is often recommended. Specifically, this entails an outline of the tasks to be evaluated at each of the various steps of the driving process. Both the new and experienced driver should be judged based on the curriculum as both will need to execute the skills required for competent vehicle operation. An example of a new driver curriculum is provided in Table 2.1. Many of these areas will overlap and will go into far greater detail during your training sessions. Progression will be determined by how the individual performs during sessions.

TABLE 2.1   Example of a Driving Curriculum.

Domain	Components
Transfer	• Wheelchair loading and storage options • Other assistive devices.
Vehicle orientation	• Primary and secondary controls • Seat adjustment, seat belt, mirror adjustment • Adaptations/modifications • Vehicle blind spots.
Starting vehicle	• Warm and cold engine.
Moving vehicle	• Shifting protocols • Start, stop, steer • Procedure for pull away, parking, turning.
Steering protocols (turning)	• Spacing/positioning • Procedure of maneuvers • Pattern development.
Range or low impact driving	• Positioning/turning/speed control • Spacing vision • Scanning skills • Parking/backing.
Moderate impact (light traffic)	• Spacing protocols "2 second rule" • Vision/scanning/lead time • Tracing/positioning • Right of way/intersection identification • Road law/signage.
High density (city driving)	• Lane use/passing • Scanning procedure • Speed control/braking/acceleration/deceleration • Diagonal parking/parallel parking • Right of way/pedestrians.
Highway driving	• Entry/exit • Passing • Speed control/cruise control • Spacing/vision • Tolls.
Weather adjustments	• 2 Second rule • Vision/glare • Skid control/evasive maneuvers • Transmission selection/speed control.
Road test skills	• 3 points Turns • Backing • Parallel parking • Stop sign protocols reviewed.
Basic maintenance	• Gas, oil, coolant • Tires • Wipers/lights.

In addition to considering the tasks being evaluated and trained, it is also important to consider the routes on which the training is being conducted. The selected routes should be reliable in the sense that, when used for specific goals, these goals will be addressed within the route. Routes commonly begin in low density environments and build upward from that point. As the traffic densities increase, it is important to include areas called "outs" as returns to less demanding situations. These "outs" will be beneficial when students become overwhelmed or if road conditions on a given day are not conducive to training goals or needs. Examples of areas to include in developing routes and symptoms are summarized in Table 2.2.

Critical Points During Driving

As the training exercises progress, one of two things will typically occur; realization that the individual is going to succeed or realization that they will not. Each one of these has different consequences for how training should proceed.

The individual who will achieve success will need to be prepared to meet any and all state division of motor vehicle requirements. This may include licensing, license classification exams, vision testing, and meeting medical fitness criteria. Upon completion of Department of Motor Vehicle (DMV) requirements, final recommendations for adaptations and modifications will be required. Depending on the individual's vehicle needs, this list may be as small as one item or as large as 30 or more items. Mobility equipment dealers and third party payers will need the final recommendations or "prescription" in developing bids and the construction of adapted/modified vehicles.

When driving is not going to be an acceptable activity for the individual then it maybe beneficial to first consider alternative interventions that may be implemented to alleviate a deficit related to driving performance. Some examples can include:

- Vision clinic/vision therapy.
- Cognitive remediation programs.
- Physical therapy for strengthening/endurance issues.
- Wheelchair seating clinic for trunk stability and seating problems.
- Occupational therapy for visual/perceptual and functional retraining.

If the possibility exists that the individual may benefit from alternative interventions recommendations from the driver specialist can be integrated into the individual's rehabilitation treatment goals. In fact, many are recommended prior to BTW aspects.

When all avenues have been exhausted and driving is just not an appropriate activity a conference with family members should be conducted. Preparation ahead of time, including preparing alternate transportation options, can help make these often difficult meeting less stressful for all involved. Offer ideas for alternative means of transportation such as mass transit, county Para-transit, Red Cross, and church groups. These possibilities, while not ideal, can ease the burden of losing driving independence.

TABLE 2.2   Description of Driving Environments to Be Included in Training Route.

Driving range or parking lots	• Development of basic fundamentals/mechanics; • Familiarize student with vehicle; • Evaluate for trunk stability, endurance, vision issues, AROM, quality of movement, divided attention and spatial relations.
Residential streets	• Low density to reinforce developed fundamentals; • Increase difficulties by including uneven terrain, winding roads, crowned roads; • Right of way, that is, uncontrolled/controlled intersections, crosswalks, stop signs and lines; • Drill SIPDE factors and Smith System; • If these are first real street experiences you may spend a lot of time in this environment developing skills and confidence; • Issue with disability such as visual field cut or neglect, endurance and trunk stability will be accentuated as you move to increased levels of difficulty; • Light to moderate traffic densities will increase the demands on scanning; • Try for a lap around lower density traffic; • Work on keeping vision ahead of "seeing big picture", lane integrity, spacing (2 second rule), and lead time; • Train on 5-second mirror checks, over shoulder checks, passing skills.
City/downtown traffic	• Working with congested traffic patterns, parking, pedestrians, etc. • Traffic signs, signals, road markings, one way roads, crosswalks, and stop lines; • Be prepared for double parking, delivery vehicles, jaywalkers, signal runners, car doors opening into roadway.
Interstate/highway driving	• Merging at higher speeds, mirror use, head over shoulder checks; • Passing, speed control, deceleration; • Global awareness in mirrors and lead time scanning 2 second rule at higher speeds; • Lane integrity, lane use on multi-lane roads; • This type of driving, although demanding in some respects, is relatively easy once your student acclimates to higher speeds.
Night-time driving and inclement weather	• If you are capable of this in your program hands on is best; • If not, instruct on "2" second rule in bad weather, use of hi-beam headlamps, application time of headlamps on/off; • When blinded by oncoming lights look down and to the right-hand side of road.
Special functions	• Try to include how-to's on tolls, drive through windows, underground parking, maintenance and emergency procedures. Include as many as you can on your routes.

ADAPTIVE DRIVING DEVICES

Today, driving control adaptations for primary and secondary control systems both low (mechanical in function) and high (power assisted) technology are readily available in assisting individuals in their operation of motor vehicles. Coupled with advanced vehicle modifications, driving has never been more available than today for persons with disabilities. The next section of this chapter provides an overview of this available technology, its application and functions.

HAND-CONTROLS: ACCELERATION AND BRAKING UNITS

Individuals unable to access acceleration and braking functions with their lower extremities can utilize hand-controls. Evaluation and training on these devices is essential in developing confidence and competence within the operator. When considering purchasing a vehicle to be adapted with hand-controls, consideration must be given to the following for the easiest application; original equipment manufacturer (OEM) items; automatic transmission; power steering; and power braking. There are systems that will allow for the use of hand-controls with a standard transmission. These systems can be costly but are effective when a manual transmission vehicle is the choice or only alternative.

There are several differing operational functions available with hand-controls. All mechanical or low tech hand-controls require a "push" away from the operator for braking function. The differences lie in the activation of acceleration of which there are several options.

   a. *Push/pull hand-controls*
- Acceleration applied by pulling to driver's torso;
- Grasp enhancing orthotics available for those with a grasp compromise;
- No capacity for simultaneous activation of acceleration/braking modes;
- One of easiest controls to initially learn.

   b. *Push/right angle pull hand-controls*
- Acceleration achieved through downward push to driver's thigh and slight pull to torso;
- Must return to full up or neutral position prior to braking to avoid simultaneous acceleration/braking;
- Release of control returns lever to neutral position;
- Acceleration in this application less fatiguing than constant pull;
- Grasp enhancers available;
- Initial training on this control may be more demanding during initial trials;
- The most utilized control throughout all populations of hand-control users.

   c. *Push/twist unit*
- Motorcycle twist grip accelerator activation;
- Usually coupled with a power assist for this function;
- More costly than mechanical control;

- Requires more maintenance than mechanical controls;
- Simultaneous acceleration/braking potential.

d. *Push/rock (lever down) unit (sure grip)*
- Acceleration achieved by pulling or rocking lever downward similar to operation of a gaming slot machine;
- Simultaneous acceleration/braking potential.

e. *Floor mounted (upright) push/pull unit*
- Found in some van applications and largely spinal cord injured populations;
- Found as an "in between" for those unable to operate standard hand-controls due to decreased active range of motion (AROM) and too strong for power assisted controls (PAC) units;
- Acceleration achieved with pulling motion;
- Orthotic interfaces often utilized as population grasps are often unreliable.

f. *Power assisted control (PAC) units*
- Operation enhanced through use of secondary power source of electrical, hydraulic, pneumatic or a combination of such power sources;
- Multiple location points assist those with limited AROM;
- Requires less AROM, strength, grasp capacities, and endurance;
- Acceleration achievable through push away, pull toward or left-to-right, right-to-left activation;
- Full acceleration to full braking from 4″ to 6″ total throw;
- Available in unilever (joystick) models which mirror that of a powered wheelchair;
- Multiple orthotic interfaces available.

Primary controls for acceleration/braking function can be applied for both left and right upper extremity operation. Some units can also be applied for use with available but limited lower extremity function, however this is rare. In many instances secondary control functions such as horn, dimmer, and directionals can be easily applied to these units.

ACCELERATION/BRAKING FUNCTION ASIDE FROM HAND-CONTROLS

As already referred, primary control operation is not limited to those needing to use their upper extremities. Although less common than the primary control devices (upper extremity) a variety of devices are available for the lower extremity.

a. *Left foot (sided) acceleration*
- For those with right lower extremity impairment but intact left lower extremity;
- Floor mounted accelerator extension from OEM pedal to left side of brake pedal;

- Permanent or quick disconnect models;
- Often tandemmed with use of OEM pedal block to prevent accidental acceleration of OEM accelerator;
- Can be very demanding in training – often more difficult than hand-controls;
- Often seen in right hemiplegia or traumatic amputation diagnosis;
- Diabetic amputation situations must prescreen for prevailing neuropathy or other diabetic indicators.

b. *Accelerator/brake pedal blocks or extensions*
- For individuals of short stature or those needing relief from air bag proximity and torso;
- Block bolt to existing OEM pedals offering extension of from 1" to 4". NOT EASILY REMOVED;
- Extensions are floor mounted and offer greater range of adjustments and attach to the OEM pedals through variable length rods;
- Extensions can be quick disconnect or fold down to floor for able operator access to OEM pedals.

STEERING MODIFICATION AND ADAPTATIONS

For individuals limited in their capacities with steering functions, there are modifications and adaptations that can assist in this operation.

1. *Steering column extensions and small diameter steering wheels*
- Mostly found in van application and wheelchair drivers but can be done in sedans as well;
- For wheelchair drivers, enhances access to an appropriate position in the driver's station;
- Adjustable columns can be extended, shortened, and offset left or right;
- Plane of the steering wheel can be moved from vertical to horizontal with left or right tilt;
- Coupled with smaller diameter steering wheels (4" to 14") and reductions in steering resistances, these systems help compensate for those with limited AROM and strength.

2. *Reduced steering efforts*
- Scaling factory effort steering at 100% effort;
- Zero or minimal effort =20% or less of factory power steering efforts;
- Reduction can be achieved through column modification, steering hear modification, and power steering box modification;
- Newer add-on digital systems interface with vehicle computer, system computer, and sensors;
- Decrease in diameter of steering wheel increases steering resistance which often indicates the need for modification;
- Reduction in steering resistance indicates need for a back-up or auxiliary steering system;

- This system provides for steering function in the case of system or vehicle failure;
- Can be electric or electric/hydraulic and is found in both van and sedan applications.

3. *Foot operated steering*
   - Applied in situations where upper extremities are not available for steering function;
   - Operates in conjunction with reduction of effort and back-up steering systems;
   - In majority of applications, left lower extremity operates floor mounted steering disc while right lower extremity operates OEM acceleration/ braking functions;
   - Often requires the remounting of all secondary controls which are normally operated by upper extremities.

4. *Steering assistive device*

The use of a steering assistive device will allow the operator complete access to all steering requirements (including evasive maneuvers) while utilizing a singular extremity. These devices are often utilized in applications including hand-controls or a paralysis or amputation of one of the upper extremities.

   a. *Spinner knob/single post grasp*
      - Requires functional grasp;
      - When limited AROM present utilized in conjunction with small diameter wheels and reduced steering efforts.
   b. *Bi-pin*
      - Often found in spinal cord injury where wrists and tendonitis are present;
      - Two posts fit across palm and back of hand;
      - Wrist flexion and extension required.
   c. *Tri-pin*
      - Three upright posts – two support wrist and third fits in the palm;
      - Applied where grasp is unreliable or non-functional;
      - Quadraplegia and a limited grasp endurance.
   d. *Palm grasp*
      - Limited grasp function and endurance populations;
      - Requires wrist pronation and some reliable grasp.
   e. *Custom splints and orthotics*
      - When commonly manufactured devices do not meet needs, custom fit units can be utilized;
      - Must be independent in access and removal to be considered;
      - Most often constructed by rehab or prosthetic engineer or mobility equipment manufacturer.

PRIMARY AND SECONDARY CONTROL DEVICES

When drivers are unable to access primary and secondary devices, these can be relocated within their AROM and/or modified so they can be activated via remote. Those controls that may be required while the vehicle is in motion include; dimmer, horn, directional signals, wiper/washer, cruise control. Those controls not requiring access while moving include; ignition, gear selector, climate controls, headlamps, radio, parking brake, windows, door locks, mirror. Controls other than vehicle controls requiring a remote can include; wheelchair securement system, steering or braking back-up systems, power headrest, etc. Low tech would include dash extensions and adapted OEM controls to meet the driver's needs. High tech will normally consist of electronic; interfaces utilizing console configurations with membrane pressure switches and may also include; toggle, extended toggle, rocker, and button switching. Scan or auditory and voice activation controls are also available.

OTHER TECHNOLOGIES

There are several other types of adaptations that allow the driver's independent entry/egress to the driving scenario. Some are very simple machine type devices and some are complex, power assisted units. Whether simple mechanical or complex electric, these devices all serve a singular purpose; allowing for independent access to the community through driving.

The following is a brief synopsis of several differing adaptations and levels of technology. When in doubt of the need or availability of assistive driving adaptations and modifications, contact a Rehabilitation Driving Professional who can answer your questions or direct you to someone who can.

a. *Transfer assistive devices*
   - Transfer boards for independent transfer to/from vehicle;
   - Transfer straps and overhead grab bars.
b. *Grasp enhancers*
   - Key bars and grasps allowing for key manipulation;
   - Generic or customized to person's needs;
   - Eliminate need for costly high tech systems.
c. *Directional/gear selector adaptations*
   - Crossovers bring functions to opposite side of OEM secondary to impaired limb;
   - Extensions bring within driver's AROM on the same side as OEM unit;
   - Low tech solutions to potentially high tech/high cost problems.
d. *Parking brake*
   - Manual extension for application with LUE;
   - Power parking brake when unable to apply OEM or manual extension;

- Some high tech acceleration/braking adaptations reduce power parking brake as part of installation and safety reasons.

e. *Wheelchair loading assistive devices*
- Cartop wheelchair carriers for those transferring into a sedan but unable to load their chair manually requires a folding frame into manual wheelchair;

TABLE 2.3   Considerations for Van Modifications.

Domain	Considerations
Entry/egress systems	• Power operated door openers for sliding or swing out doors; • Operation of semi- or fully-automatic ramps and lefts; • Operated through the use of remote control, magnetic switching systems, and/or weatherproof toggle switches, mainly dependent on client's capabilities; • Lifts consist of platform or rotary; • Face forward entry or rotary lefts and are parallel to vehicle; • Back onto platform lefts perpendicular to vehicle; • Available for both full size and minivans but not applicable to all makes and models; • Ramps consist of both fold out and pocket stored and are found in conjunction with chassis kneeling systems on minivan; • Egress clearances: (rotary left 3′–5′; platform lift 5′–9′; minivan ramp 5′–9′).
Clearance modification	• For door opening clearance and access to driving station at appropriate vision line; • Drop floor conversions: (full size 2″–14″ drop floor; minivan 10″–12″ drop floor); • Can cover cargo, driver and/or passenger areas; • Certain makes and models are available to this type conversion (see DRP for application); • Side or rear entry modifications available; • Reverse power elevator available for those needing to be elevated from drop or stock floor heights to driving vision line; • Drop power pan available where a full area drop is not desired. Wheelchair width issues apply; • Sport top or raised roof to increase interior clearances without dropping floor; • Raised doorway entry to allow clear access through the doorway.
Wheelchair and occupant restraint systems	• Manual 4-point belt systems for transport situations 4-point mount on chair and floor; • Powered or automatic tie-downs for driver and transport applications (requires bracketry permanently attached to wheelchair) 4 or 5 points of mount on wheelchair to 1 or 2 points on floor; • Transfer wheelchair tie-down used to secure wheelchair once client transfers to a power seat (this can be powered or manual).

- Truck or hatch loaders for those unable to load their chairs whether power or manual or their scooters;
- May require some disassembling of the mobility assistive device;
- Client must be capable of ambulating to driver station and/or independent transfer in these applications;
- Can eliminate the need for costly van adaptations and modifications.

VAN TRANSPORTATION

In many cases, a standard vehicle is not a suitable option for individuals. The most common choices include a full size van or minivan. In considering this, several factors must be evaluated and several options are available.

Choice of vehicle will greatly rely on the size of the client as coupled with their mobility assistive device. Interior clearances such as floor to top of client's head and client's vision line must be addressed when considering proper vehicle and vehicle modifications. The detail of these considerations will largely be affected by whether the client will drive from their power or manual wheelchair or transfer into a power seat. It is imperative that individuals seeking a van for mobility receive a comprehensive driving evaluation, insuring the appropriate choices in this complex process. Table 2.3 summarizes some primary considerations for van modifications.

CONCLUSIONS

This has been a very brief overview of some of the assistive technology available in aiding persons with disabilities to operate motor vehicles. Indeed, an entire book could be written regarding all available technologies and their applications in the field. The DRS and CDRS who conduct comprehensive driver evaluation and training programs are most knowledgeable in the technology sector. Also consultation with a mobility equipment dealer/installer serves as an excellent source of information regarding this highly specialized area. Because of their expertise in the manufacturing and installation of modifications and adaptations, the mobility dealer may have insights that the DRS/CDRS may not have knowledge of. It is for this reason that the DRS/CDRS and mobility equipment dealer must work as a team in providing the utmost in professional services for our clients and their highly specific needs.

3

DRIVING CONSULTATION AND INTERVENTION

ROSAMOND GIANUTSOS

Driving consultation is a clinical evaluation and counseling service designed to help at-risk drivers in deciding whether, when, where, and how to drive. In most societies, driving is subject to state licensure; however, there is a need to recognize that each driver is the ultimate licensor. Each time the driver puts the key in the ignition, there is an implicit judgment: I can handle this task safely. Driving consultation is advocated as a service to help keep at-risk drivers safely in the driver's seat, even when that means deciding to give up the keys. By extension, where this is not feasible, driving consultation supports families and communities by identifying what has to be done. Driving consultation is concerned not only with changing driving behavior, but also with helping individuals come to terms with those changes. The range of available services is broad and one size does not fit all. What is envisioned here are tiered services that are independent of the departments of motor vehicles, though guided by the laws of the jurisdictions they serve (Janke & Eberhard, 1998; De Raedt & Ponjaert-Kristoffersen, 2001).

The last decade has seen a gratifying increase in attention to driving, both with the growth of driver rehabilitation and with research on driver evaluation. This chapter is an attempt to draw our attention to the clinical, human service aspects of consulting with at-risk drivers, would-be drivers, and their families. This chapter is a distillation of experiences in: (1) working with survivors of brain injury who wish to resume driving; (2) training clinicians who are running or setting up driver rehabilitation units; (3) developing and coordinating research on two computerized driving advisement protocols (Driving Advisement System and Elemental Driving Simulator (EDS)) and, like most people in our society; and

(4) being a resource for the members of my family who have had to address these issues. This last aspect has reinforced my appreciation of the need to address driving effectively, with great sensitivity, and often ingenuity.

Who are the cognitively at-risk drivers and would-be drivers? And to whom do they turn for help? In general, individuals fall into three broad classes: (1) youth with disabling conditions which have kept them from mainstream driver education, (2) drivers with acquired brain injury who wish to resume, and (3) older drivers who are undergoing cognitive changes. While experienced driver reha- bilitation specialists report that the first group typically presents the greatest chal- lenges, the needs of the youth with disabling conditions are more for evaluation and training. For the present discussion the focus will be on the persons who have established themselves as drivers at some time in the past who need counseling or consultation, as well as evaluation – the second and third groups above. Those drivers who have sustained a brain injury, such as a stroke or brain trauma, have been forced to stop driving suddenly, are usually under medical supervision and desire to resume driving, possibly with physical and sensory disability, in addition to the cognitive problems caused by brain injury. Their general status may continue to improve, or at least stay the same, as recovery goes on. Within a rehabilitation context, for the persons with acquired brain injury, there is an increased likelihood that driving will be raised by the treating team, although it has not yet become a standard of care in brain injury rehabilitation.

The other subgroup of concern includes those older drivers with age associated cognitive changes which have been progressing gradually. While they may have changed the frequency and type of driving, they continue to enjoy the privilege of deciding when to take the wheel. Interestingly enough, most experienced driv- ers – including the members of these two constituencies – express considerable confidence in their ability to drive safely. For most adult drivers, driving is not just about safe mobility. It has become synonymous with independence and feel- ings of competency. Older people will say, "after all, I have been driving for ... years" as if experience alone matters, and not physical and mental function. Many may quietly limit their driving and some avail themselves of mature driving courses. Rarely, however, are they seeking further help. For this group concerns are usually raised by others, mostly family members. These family members may risk family harmony and take matters into their own hands. Some will stop riding with the person, but otherwise ignore the problem – preserving family harmony, if not safety. Others seek outside help, usually turning to their primary care doctor, or if available, a relevant specialist, such as a geriatrician, a neurologist, or an eye doctor. One suggestion for older persons is to introduce driver consultation as part of retirement planning, with an opportunity to obtain a baseline and to urge people to plan for the day when they will no longer be able to drive.

This chapter is intended to identify the important clinical issues for clinicians and for the driver rehabilitation specialists to whom individuals and families may turn for driving consultation.

LEGAL CONSIDERATIONS

One of the first services within the realm of driving consultation is advising clients and colleagues of their legal obligations. Based on a survey conducted by Pidikiti and Novack (1991), it has been reported that health care providers are often uninformed or underinformed about the applicable laws regarding driving. Yet, the laws are very specific and clinicians should make every effort to obtain copies of the specific state laws and policies. One resource for this information, is available through the American Medical Association (AMA), which in 2003 put together the "Physicians guide to assessing and counseling older drivers" (http://www.ama-assn.org/ama/pub/category/10791.html). This free guide, which is available in both electronic and print copies include a comprehensive review of the literature on driving and older drivers, and summarizes laws and policy for each of the 50 states. Information from such resources can be summarized and developed into a pamphlet or brief statement about local regulations to serve as a useful way to assure that all concerned have the correct information.

In addition to information about state laws, information about specific reporting laws should be provided, to help inform all individuals about clinical obligations and expectations. Again, much variability exists from state to state regarding reporting. While in some jurisdictions there is a mandatory reporting policy; in others reporting by concerned health care providers is discouraged by a lack of immunity from lawsuits asserting a violation of the patient's privacy. As Antrim and Engum (1989) explain, the biggest legal risk is doing nothing. If a rehabilitation facility is offering services designed to promote physical recovery and community re-entry, they should know that their clients will attempt to resume driving, even if they don't ask. Furthermore, recommendations need to be put in writing with documentation that the patient received the information.

An information pamphlet, such as described above, serves to introduce the issue of driving, so that it will be addressed as part of health care delivery. In a study of driving after stroke (Fisk et al., 1997), 48% did not receive advice about driving and 87% said they received no evaluation. Rehabilitation health care providers are often astounded to learn that certain patients have, or intend to, resume driving. There are good reasons to raise the issue of driving early on in rehabilitation, well before actual driving would be possible. Addressing this issue early allows the individual to make plans, including whether to fix or sell the car, or suspend the insurance to save money. It puts the would-be driver on notice that this issue is included in the rehabilitation agenda. In sum, a regularized proactive approach to driving can be beneficial to both providers and individuals seeking services.

MEDICAL CLEARANCE

Much of the legal burden is placed on physicians and optometrists regarding medical competency to drive. Although some guidelines exist for different conditions (such as recommendations by the Association of Driver Rehabilitation Specialists), it is not always clear that practitioners have this information (Pidikiti & Novack, 1991).

More commonly, doctors will see forms which they may be asked to fill out for Motor Vehicles. These define the minimum medical criteria for licensure, which vary from state to state. For example, for vision there is usually a standard of best corrected acuity and possibly visual field. A broader view of the health care provider's responsibility would suggest that the medical consultant should identify all those medical conditions that could affect a person's driving, especially those which are episodic in nature, or hidden to direct observation. An example in vision would be a loss of binocularity. While this does not disqualify one from an ordinary operator's license, it could affect driving in predictable ways, for example, judgment of distances. In the case described below, the loss of binocularity could have contributed to the motor vehicle crashes. Formal studies have shown that glaucoma and cataracts, conditions common in older drivers, more than double crash risk compared to age-matched controls (Owsley et al., 1998; Owsley et al., 1999; Wood & Mallon, 2001). There is a need for comprehensive driver consultation that makes the connection between medical conditions and driving.

> A clinical example is a patient with three injury-producing motor vehicle crashes in ten years. Two of the crashes resulted in brain injury, including the third, in which she was rear-ended when she stopped suddenly for an unexpected signal. In a routine rehabilitative optometric evaluation, she was discovered to have advanced, previously undiagnosed glaucoma. She had lost almost all useable vision in one eye. The other eye was showing signs of glaucoma, but still had the requisite acuity and visual field for licensure. Upon learning this diagnosis, her psychologist, neuropsychologist and optometrist all urged her to stop driving immediately, pending further evaluation and treatment, including resolution of the cognitive problems caused by her injuries. However, when she saw an ophthalmologist for her glaucoma, she asked if she could drive and reportedly was given a favorable reply. This advice related narrowly to the legal visual pre-requisites for driving. This patient has resumed driving.

As desirable as it may be for physicians and allied health professionals to reach out to their patients regarding driving, most of them do not have expertise in driving. Even if they are asked for an opinion, they should make the limits of that opinion clear. Not only did the ophthalmologist in the case above appear to interpret the issue of driving narrowly within the guidelines for vision, but also did not take into consideration cognitive problems which could be expected to influence driving competency. It is quite possible that the patient, eager to resume driving, only heard that portion of the ophthalmologist's advice that bore on her satisfaction of the legal requirements for driving.

NON-INDIVIDUALIZED APPROACHES: GENERAL RESOURCES

A multi-tiered approach to Driving Consultation would include informational services which are not individually tailored. These approaches are especially appropriate for older drivers who are not known to have sustained a brain injury or stroke. Excellent informational materials have been developed by such organizations such as the AAA Foundation for Traffic Safety, for instance, "Drivers 55+: Test Your Own Performance" (Malfetti & Winter, 1991), also www.aaa-foundation.org/pdf/driver55.pdf, and "How to Help and Older Driver" (Malfetti & Winter, 1992), also www.aaafoundation.org/pdf/ODlarge.pdf; and the American Association of Retired Persons (AARP) "Older Driver Skill Assessment and Resource Guide (Creating Mobility Choices)"(American Association of Retired Persons, 1992). These organizations and others are developing fine web-based tools. Good starting places are www.drivers.com, the frequently asked questions page of the "55 Alive" program: www.aarp.org/55alive/faq.html and www.cogre-hab.com/tools/drivertools.php3. Further, older driver issues are often addressed by the popular media, although these often accentuate the negative aspects. For many older drivers these services suffice to allow them to make the necessary adjustments to their driving.

For many years, the AARP has sponsored the "55 Alive" peer-led driver safety ("defensive driving") courses, which offer information and peer support. It has been alleged that defensive driving courses are sought out by conscientious concerned drivers who, being predisposed to their contents, don't need them. Regardless, the point is that these resources are available and may be all that is necessary for some individuals and those concerned about them to make appropriate decisions.

INDIVIDUALIZED APPROACHES: DRIVING CONSULTATION

Inevitably, however, there will be others who need more specific and individualized attention. Much attention has been paid by the National Highway Traffic Safety Administration to the older driver. An extensive report (Staplin et al., 1999) contains a model driver screening and evaluation program (see also, www.nhtsa. dot.gov/people/injury/olddrive/safe/index.htm) that is offered as a means to determine the need for individualized driving consultation. In addition, the Association for Driver Rehabilitation Specialists (www.driver-ed.org) also provides lists of symptoms that are thought to be indicative of the need for an individualized driver evaluation (e.g., driving too slow/inappropriate driving speed, doesn't observe signs). Finally, certain diagnoses are thought to raise the question of individualized driver consultation. These are addressed in the other chapters of this book.

Generally, candidates for individualized driving consultation are those who are cognitively or behaviorally at-risk, usually because of some known or suspected brain dysfunction. Persons with psychiatric diagnoses are also likely to benefit from individualized driving consultation, although this area has been underdeveloped. For instance, it is known that adults with attention deficit disorder have poorer driving records than their age-matched peers (Barkley et al., 1993; Barkley et al., 1996).

Individualized driving consultation is designed to focus on two categories of need: (1) conditions which impair the driver's ability to evaluate their own performance, for example, severe memory impairment, lack of insight, behavioral disturbance, or loss of contact with reality; and (2) conditions which by their nature are hard to evaluate subjectively. In this latter category fall many kinds of neurologically based visual impairments, including field loss and loss of binocularity.

It is apparent that many people who need driving consultation are unlikely to seek it out unless prompted to do so by their families, health care providers, or to meet legal requirements. This is especially true for older drivers who might expect that the driving consultation would threaten their independence. It is therefore, important for the providers of driving consultation to have something positive to offer, even if it is information about reduced fare public transit cards and other programs which offer alternative mobility.

WHAT ARE THE PRACTICAL CONSIDERATIONS?

Usually one of the first questions is, *"Is it covered by insurance?"* The answer has to be: "Don't count on it." Driving consultation can be considered a medical service when there is a medical diagnosis of brain impairment. However, there is no procedure code explicitly designed for individualized driving consultation. If the driver rehabilitation specialist is a licensed health care provider, for example, occupational therapist or neuropsychologist, it is possible that the evaluation process may fall under evaluation of activities of daily living or as a neurobehavioral status exam. To date, it remains unknown how utilization of this service is affected by costs. When one considers the expense of driving, estimated by the American Automobile Association at between 3000 and 6000 per year (www. ouraaa.com/news/library/drivingcost/), a few hundred dollars for driving consultation doesn't seem unreasonable. On the other hand, given the safety implications for both the patient and others, it would be an enlightened policy for the costs of these services to be absorbed in whole or in part by society. One model would be to have it subsumed under the same umbrella as defensive driving courses, which often qualify for an insurance discount and a reduction of points.

When should driving consultation begin? Initial steps can be taken at the first hint of concern, or early in recovery from a brain injury or stroke. These steps could include "bibliotherapy," informing the individual of legal requirements and encouraging them to seek a professional evaluation prior to resuming driving. When a brain injured driver becomes physically able to resume driving and has access to a vehicle, it is important to ascertain the individual's intentions and desires. While it may seem pointless to do an evaluation when there is a high likelihood of failure, it may be necessary if the person plans to resume driving. In one clinical case, an older man inquired about an early evaluation, stating: "I know I am not ready to drive, I just want to know how far off I am." When there is a family member, usually a spouse, who is in a position to control the would-be driver's access to a car, it is important to obtain that person's agreement to go along with your recommendations, even if it means driving resumption.

Who is qualified to perform an individualized driving consultation? In the United States there are nearly 300 Certified Driver Rehabilitation Specialists (CDRS) comprised mostly of Occupational Therapists, but also many Driver Educators and a few Psychologists. These individuals are certified through the Association for Driver Rehabilitation Specialists, which has a web site through which one might find a CDRS (www.driver-ed.org). Many rehabilitation centers have one or more therapists prepared to offer driving assessment and consultation. Some states have evaluation units within the Department of Motor Vehicles, for example, Connecticut which has had a Handicapped Driver Unit. Though mostly intended to serve persons with physical disabilities, this unit will pick up a candidate driver for an evaluation/training session in the individual's neighborhood.

The evaluation of physical disability and prescription of adaptive devices for driving is a developing specialty within Occupational Therapy (Beatson & Gianutsos, 2000; Pierce, 1996). While these conditions warrant referral to a driver rehabilitation center that has the equipment and expertise for adaptive driving, evaluation of cognitive and behavioral issues, as will be discussed here, is important to determine if the person will be able to use the adaptive equipment safely.

THE DRIVING CONSULTATION PROCESS

The first step is to obtain a driving history and find out what kind of driving the person used to do. As your older clients will be quick to remind you, experience does make a great deal of difference. What the person says about their driving can often be revealing. A Swedish study (Lundqvist & Ronnberg, 2001) showed that success in an on-road evaluation was related to pre-morbid interest in and motivation for safe driving. Does the prospective driver show an appreciation of safety issues, both in driving and in other areas? Did they enjoy driving? What type of car did they drive and why did they pick it? What is its current mileage and condition? It is also possible to obtain information from the Department of Motor Vehicles to confirm the recent history of significant crashes and violations. If there have been recent crashes, a close analysis is recommended to determine if cognitive, behavioral, or sensory factors may have been contributory.

Next, what are the candidate driver's current needs and intentions? Does the person say they "have to drive," or will driving be an option? Can they limit when and where to drive? Will the person be pressured to drive in order to work or to respond to externally imposed requirements or schedules? It is important to find out what significant others think about the person's driving. What is the basis for their concerns? It can also be revealing to ask the person what they think others will say.

Frequently people will say that they have to drive, and this assertion needs to be challenged. It is based on certain assumptions, such as living in a particular place or engaging in a particular job. Granted, as stated earlier, our society has been designed for driving. Nevertheless, in theory, if not in practice, driving should always be an option, a conscious choice.

Medical background and prognosis are necessary, especially if there are conditions which are episodic in nature (seizures, coronary problems, and sleep disorder), likely to get worse (e.g., degenerative diseases), or whose symptoms might not be evident upon examination.

ASSESSMENT: THE EDS

The major division in the assessment is between the on-road and the off-road components. Details of the on-road and off-road assessment are provided in other chapters. However, this chapter will introduce an additional off-road tool that can inform the overall driver consultation. That is, the Elemental Driving Simulator (EDS) (Gianutsos, 1994; Gianutsos & Beattie, 1992); which uses a personal computer with a small steering wheel, turn signal and pedals, illustrated in Figure 3.1.

The EDS incorporates the principles delineated below. First as with any psychological test, psychometric standards are essential for any assessment of driving capacity. It is remarkable how many widely used procedures for driver rehabilitation have little or no psychometric documentation. Most procedures developed in the last decade have improved in this regard. Psychometric development means, first, that there must be an appropriate norm group, in this case representing the broad spectrum of drivers. The EDS does not use age-based norms, as the standard of comparison is the performance of other drivers. Second, the measures must have demonstrable reliability, so that essentially the same results would be obtained upon re-testing at another time, with an alternative assessment or a different examiner. Third, the procedures must have proven (empirical) validity to show that they relate to driving safety and mobility. For instance, in a study with Occupational Therapist Amy Campbell, we found a significant relationship of EDS performance with the outcome of a road test (see Figure 3.2).

However, for clinical effectiveness perhaps most important, is that the procedures have apparent or "face" validity. They must look to the examinee like they relate to driving. Finally, the assessment used for driver consultation must address metacognitive functions, that is, the ability to assess one's own abilities and the consequent decisions about when and how to drive. The importance of this is obvious if the entire process is viewed as one of determining if the individual remains capable of being the "ultimate licensor" of her or his own driving. One strategy is to ask for estimates of performance relative to other drivers, as illustrated in Figure 3.3.

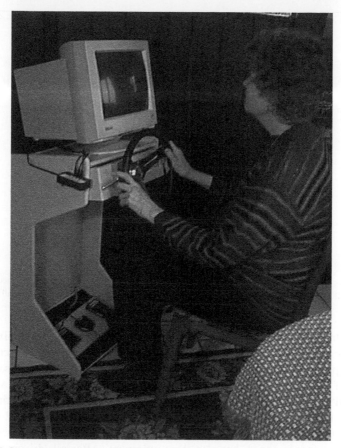

FIGURE 3.1   Participant using the EDS.

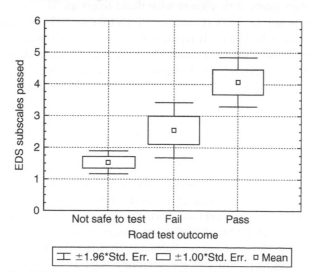

FIGURE 3.2   EDS and road test outcome, based on an analysis of clinical records in a comprehensive driver rehabilitation program. Courtesy of Amy Campbell, OTR, CDRS.

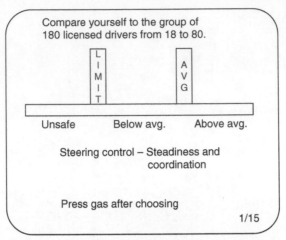

FIGURE 3.3   EDS self-appraisal task screen. The examinee uses the steering wheel to move the marker horizontally to the spot on the line where they believe their present abilities fall.

To address these various points, the EDS was designed to measure six aspects of driving and includes six "Self-Appraisal" items (see Table 3.1). Accordingly, the self-appraisals can then be scaled (i.e., an "average" self-appraisal is assigned a score of 100 and a self-appraisal at the "limit" of safety is assigned a 70) and compared to norm-referenced performance scores. So if a person says their reaction time is slightly above average, and their actual performance is 2 standard deviation units below average (about the 2.5 percentile), one would question not only their response speed, but also their judgment. After all, drivers can only drive within their limits, if they know what those limits are.

One study using the EDS (Gianutsos & DeLibero, 1999) focused on self-appraisals, (Table 3.2) driver self-report (ratings of how they would drive in difficult situations), and EDS performance. All participants were currently driving and had no relevant neurological diagnosis. Some were students in their 20s and 30s and some were older drivers from a community center, average age 76 years. The EDS performance of these two groups, along with that of the standard EDS normative sample is shown in Figure 3.4.

While the young adults performance on the EDS matched the norms, the older drivers performed almost 2 standard deviation units below the norms, that is, close to the clinical cutoff of the EDS. These data suggest that EDS performance may be associated with age associated cognitive changes.

More interesting were the findings for Self-Appraisal and Driver Self-Report. The older drivers' gave self-appraisals which were slightly, but statistically significantly, higher than the broad EDS norm group. In contrast, their self-reports, as well as their performance, were substantially lower than the younger adult drivers. While self-appraisal did not correlate with EDS performance, there was a very high correlation between EDS performance and Driver Self-Report

TABLE 3.1   Aspects of Driving Measured by the EDS.

Aspect	Driving example	Self-appraisal	EDS performance
Steering control Steadiness and coordination	Narrow two way streets Mountain roads Parking Narrowed construction lanes	Eye-hand coordination; ability to steer accurately and steadily	Steering standard deviation averaged across all three phases. Standard deviation is the variability in deviation from center on the roadway
Reaction speed Simple reaction time	Sudden presence of unambiguous hazard Emergency response	Basic response time; little thinking or decision-making involved	Median reaction time* for Phase 2 (WATCHING FOR "FRED"); mean reaction time is an alternate measure
Visual field Aware of the far left and far right	Aware of vehicles in other lanes on highway Pedestrians, cyclists entering roadway Intersection events	Consistency of response to both sides of the display	Difference between Right and Left Median Response on Phases 2 and 3
Adjusting Quickly and easily to changes	Unexpected (other) driver error Rental or borrowed car Driving on the other side of the road Construction zone changes Emergency sirens heard Accident has just occurred Weather changes (e.g., hail)	Processing efficiency in complex situations; ability to respond flexibly, as in an emergency or new situation	Median reaction time* for Phase 3 (HAZARD AVOIDANCE); mean reaction time is an alternate measure
Self-control Resist the urge to act quickly when more thought is required	Deciding when to pass another car Deciding when to merge onto highway (Not) making turns/lane changes at the last minute (Not) advancing when other traffic does, even though they have the light and you don't (Not) advancing on delayed green	Ability to refrain from, or to retract, and action, such as not slamming on the brakes on an icy road	Erroneous signal responses (%) in Phase 3
Consistency Driving in the same way	(Not) accelerating and decelerating rapidly (Not) making frequent lane changes (Not) letting emotions influence your driving (avoiding road rage) (Not) having good days and bad days	Predictability of driver's behavior to other drivers, ability to sustain a level of performance; regularity of performance	Difference between mean and median reaction time in all test phases;** standard deviation of response times is an alternate index

TABLE 3.2   Driver Self-Report

"How" items	
Signal	Intentions and check the rear when changing lanes
Seat belt	Wear a seat belt
"When" items	
In rain or fog	Drive just as much as others do
In snow or sleet	Drive just as much as others do
At night	Just as much as others do
Highways	Just as often as others do
High traffic areas	As much as others do
Unfamiliar roads	As often as others do
Trips over an hour	As often as others do

($r = 0.69$). The older drivers made statements of confidence in their abilities, but expressed caution about how they chose to drive in specific situations, for example, "I am quite capable of driving, I just choose not to take on as much as I used to." So, this normal older group appeared to be limiting their driving to a degree that was consistent with their simulator performance.

In sum, the EDS attempts to measure the following driving domains: Steering Steadiness, Simple and Complex Reaction Time, Consistency, Self-Control, and Lateral Differential Response (important because neurological injury is often lateralized). It also explicitly attempts to measure metacognition.

ASSESSMENT: OTHER CONSIDERATIONS

Generally, driving involves an integrated set of overlearned operational skills which, in the experienced driver, are performed without a great deal of conscious control. The human operator does most driving "without thinking," but is quickly able to assert fully conscious control when circumstances require it. As such, the assessment should address the efficiency and quality of these underlying operational skills, as well as the ability for controlled decision making. The first skill related to driving that people think of is reaction time; however, the assessment must go well beyond simple reaction time.

Because driving is based on this foundation of overlearned operational skills, the assessment process should allow ample opportunity for practice. No matter how much the clinical task looks like driving, it will still be different and may require some getting used to. It can be argued that how long it takes for the individual to get used to the task is not nearly so important, as their ultimate level of performance. For some, allowing the individual to have some control over how

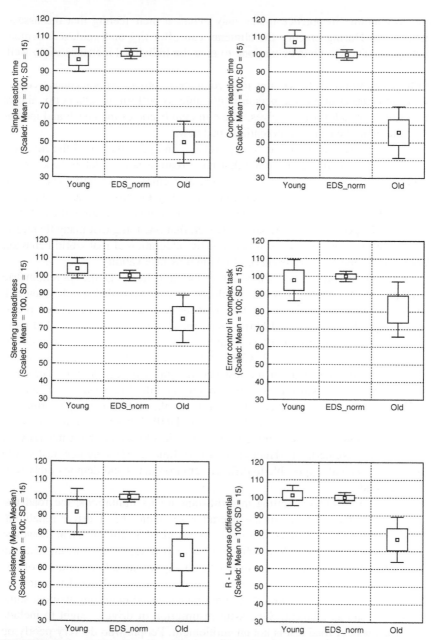

FIGURE 3.4 Performance of community residing older ($N = 19$, average age = 76 years) and young adult ($N = 20$, average age = 26) drivers compared to EDS general normative data sample ($N = 103$ drivers ranging in age from 18 to 80, average age = 37). The "whiskers" represent a two standard error confidence interval. On all measures, the older group was significantly lower than the other two groups. The average performance of the older drivers was close to the two standard deviation clinical cutoff, based on the normative sample.

long to continue in practice mode, may enhance their feeling that the assessment is fair. During practice the clinician can offer tips and guidance, demonstrating that everything is being done to give the individual a chance to do well.
If norm-referenced feedback is offered during practice, then the individual has
multiple opportunities to see how they compare to others. This feedback can be
highly motivating and if the person is not able to perform as others do, allows
the results to speak for themselves. The clinician becomes the coach and media-
tor, rather than the bearer of potentially bad news.

It is unfortunate that clinicians, researchers, and patients regard the road test
as the "gold standard," considering that most road tests completely lack formal
psychometric properties: norms, reliability, and empirical validity. The "sweat
standard" is a more apt characterization of the way most road tests work: if the
patient's driving causes the examiner to sweat (feel uncomfortable), the outcome
is likely to be poor. It has to be said, however, that one thing that many therapists
value about the road test is that it is a holistic integration of real world behavior.
Patients value the road test because of its obvious face validity.

As noted by others, an important research priority is the psychometric
development of a road test which would deserve to be called a gold standard.
It is a challenge because each setting is different. The most organized previous attempt (Forbes et al., 1975) was implemented as an advanced driving
test in New Zealand. In each test locale, extensive documentation was developed and examiners required 2 weeks training. Questions were also raised as
to the discriminatory value of the test because most people passed. There are
recent attempts to produce a psychometrically qualified on road test, including
the Washington University Road Test (Hunt et al., 1997), and a performance-
based test (Odenheimer et al., 1994). A new TRIP (Test-ride for Investigating
Practical Fitness to Drive) protocol is being developed at the University of
Gronigan, The Netherlands (Hunt et al., 1997; Tant, 2002). Any new test would
have to be practical, applicable to different environments and demonstrably reliable and valid.

In the current clinical setting, notwithstanding its limitations, the road test
is an important component in the overall assessment. Most driver rehabilitation specialists now recognize that the road test alone is not sufficient; however,
the Association for Driver Rehabilitation Specialists identifies it as an essential
component of any evaluation. Yet in practice a slightly modified variation of this
policy appears to hold greater consensus: people whose risk level warrants an
individualized driver evaluation should not be advanced to driving without some
kind of on-road assessment. Successful resumption of driving ought to include
an on-road test. A road test is not an entitlement. People who do very poorly on
the in-clinic assessment, or who exhibit behavior or attitudinal problems, may
not be tested because of safety considerations. Because road tests tend to emphasize operational skills, a person with behavioral or attitudinal problems might
perform well, even though common sense tells us that the person is not yet ready
to be driving.

Because the road test is the last step in the assessment process, it often becomes the "last word." This can be unfortunate because road tests are relatively insensitive. Further, in many cases they are conducted by driver educators who have little or no medical training or experience. It can be argued that a positive on-road result does not necessarily override a negative in-clinic evaluation. If there are sufficient concerns raised by the in-clinic results, it is a good idea for the clinician to meet with the patient and concerned others after the road test.

TIPS FOR CONVEYING THE RESULTS AND RECOMMENDATIONS

1. *Favorable outcome*: Conveying results and recommendations is not difficult when the outcome is favorable to driving. The basic message should be along the lines of: I have checked out your abilities carefully and can not find anything which makes you significantly different from other drivers. This does not guarantee that you will drive safely, only that you have the abilities to do so. Further, you have demonstrated that you understand the risks and responsibilities of driving.

2. *Borderline outcome*: More often than not, there will be some cautions or limitations that you would recommend. If this is the case, avoid presenting the findings as a "contingent pass" unless you are comfortable with the possibility that the contingencies will be ignored. It is helpful if there are others present for the discussion of such contingencies, especially if these others will be in a position to promote adherence to the limitations or follow through on the recommendations, for example, supervised driving, lessons, etc.

In situations where the person's performance is borderline, it is important to state this conclusion clearly. If you think the person's abilities have changed, tell them. Emphasize that in order to be safe, they will have to drive differently. Here the clinician has to judge whether the person is likely to modify their driving. For people with concrete thinking, specific guidelines will need to be developed. And, of course, it should be stated that the less driving the person does, the better. If there is someone else who could do the driving, encourage the person to defer to the other driver. The guidelines should specify if rides can be given to others, and if so, how much information should be given to prospective passengers (a variation on informed consent).

3. *Progressive diagnosis*: When there is a possibility that the person's condition will vary, or, especially, worsen, the basic message has to be, "The question is not whether to give up driving, but when and how." We would all like to be able to continue to drive until the very moment that we cross the mythical threshold into the unsafe category. However, given the possibility of an error in decision-making, clearly, it is better to make the error of stopping too early, rather than too late. The idea is to start the person thinking about disengaging from driving, and finding alternatives. Further, it is important to plan for reappraisal,

both within a given time frame, and if problems arise. If possible, identify benchmarks and warning signals for the individual and their families.

4. *Unfavorable outcome*: Finally, when the person does not do well and you are convinced that they are not safe to drive at the present time, you must state this opinion clearly. If you think there is a chance, or even a likelihood, that they will never be able to drive safely, you can introduce this idea gently by saying, "You need to consider the possibility that you may never be able to drive safely. Your future plans, for example, where to live, vocational directions, should not be dependent on your being able to drive." In some cases, individuals will request a "second chance" to improve their performance. Unless there was a technical glitch or other factor which prevented the assessment from being valid, it is a good idea to defer further evaluation for 3 to 6 months.

Finally, the result of the clinical assessment needs to be summarized in writing, as well as in a face-to-face discussion, in terms that the patient and concerned others can understand. Agreement is reached before beginning the assessment as to the disposition of this report. Some facilities require the patient to give pre-consent for the report to be sent to the Department of Motor Vehicles, if the results are not positive. I do not favor such a policy, as it may discourage someone from getting the assessment, for fear that the issue of their driving would be taken out of their hands.

INTERVENTIONS

What can you offer the people who do not initially earn your endorsement of resumption of independent driving? An important first distinction, is to differentiate those individuals who have a realistic chance of resuming driving and those for whom your goal is that they should come to understand and accept why they can't resume driving. In the latter case, you can attempt to identify specific prerequisites that the person can work on.

1. *Driving lessons*: Without doubt, individual driving lessons can be useful. This can be accomplished either with a driver specialist, or in some cases with a local driving instructor. In both cases, but in particular with the latter, it is important to work with the driving instructor to ensure that concerns about cognition, judgment, and behavior are integrated into the lessons.

2. *Supervised driving*: In some cases, it may be beneficial to become actively involved in managing an individuals' driving activity to ensure the most appropriately gradual resumption of driving. For example, an individual can be asked to keep a written log of every trip, including anything unusual. Driving may begin with only specific places on previously agreed-upon routes. Monthly on-road drives and re-evaluation of progress can help to monitor if improvement is being seen. This can include a review not only of specific driving behaviors, but also route selection and/or identify safer routes to the same destination. In addition, driving skills under different conditions, such as night time driving, can be gradually introduced and evaluated.

3. *Promoting alternate mobility*: It is important to encourage the use of alternate mobility, such as may be available. This can be presented as a backup for driving or as practice in many of the independent mobility activities on which driving depends. Often, it is necessary to teach the person how to use public transit, including arranging for schedules and tickets. Independent pedestrian mobility is essential.

In some communities there are innovative programs for alternate safe mobility, such as the Independent Transportation Network in Portland Maine (http://www.itninc.org), "a dignified, independent transportation solution for seniors." The USAA (http://www.usaa.com), which offers auto insurance to the military community, has a special on-call car service.

4. *Active passenger technique*: The active passenger technique consists of having the prospective driver sitting in the front passenger seat offering commentary about the driving situation. It is a variation on commentary driving, a method used for years by driver educators. The task can be structured, for instance, by having the person monitor for certain kinds of signs. Or, there can be challenging by questions, such as "What is the current speed limit?" or "Who has the right of way?" The comments of the active passenger can be illuminating, earning confidence or undermining it, as the case may be.

5. *Computerized exercises*: Exercises ostensibly are intended to build and strengthen abilities. For example, one study (Klavora et al., 1995) shows promise for Dynavision training. However, we have no guarantee that they will do so, or that there will be generalization to driving. Regardless, exercises do serve to educate the individual on the scope and limits of their abilities. So, doing exercises is potentially a win–win proposition: the abilities may improve, but so will the person's understanding of the limits of their abilities. This understanding is the foundation for metacognition and the application of judgment to driving.

CONCLUSION

The take-home message is the clinical aspect of driving consultation. In a society like ours, driving has become essential to independence and the loss of driving privileges has much personal significance. Driving needs to be a focus of active rehabilitative attention, coordinated by Driver Rehabilitation Specialists. The emphasis should be on safe mobility for life (to borrow a phrase which is the title of a major initiative of the US Department of Transportation), even when that means independent community mobility without driving.

REFERENCES

American Association of Retired Persons (1992). *Older Driver Skill Assessment and Resource Guide: Creating Mobility Choices*. Washington, DC: AARP.

Antrim, J. M., & Engum, E. S. (1989). The driving dilemma and the law: Patients' striving for independence vs. public safety. *Cognit. Rehabil.*, 7(2 (March/April)), 16–19.

Barkley, R. A., Guevremont, D. C., Anastopoulos, A. D., DuPaul, G. J., & Shelton, T. L. (1993). Driving-related risks and outcomes of attention deficit hyperactivity disorder in adolescents and young adults: A 3- to 5-year follow-up survey. *Pediatrics*, 92(2), 212–218.

Barkley, R. A., Murphy, K. R., & Kwasnik, D. (1996). Motor vehicle driving competencies and risks in teens and young adults with attention deficit hyperactivity disorder. *Pediatrics*, 98(6), 1089–1095.

Beatson, C. J., & Gianutsos, R. (2000). Personal transportation: The vital link to independence. In: M. Grabois, S. J. Garrison, K. A. Hart, & L. D. Lehmkuhl (Eds.), *Physical medicine and rehabilitation: The complete approach* (pp. 777–802). Malden, MA: Blackwell Science, Inc.

De Raedt, R., & Ponjaert-Kristoffersen, I. (2001). Short cognitive/neuropsychological test battery for first-tier fitness-to-drive assessment of older adults. *Clin. Neuropsychol.*, 15(3), 329–336.

Fisk, G. D., Owsley, C., & Pulley, L. V. (1997). Driving after stroke: Driving exposure, advice, and evaluations. *Arch. Phys. Med. Rehabil.*, 78, 1338–1345.

Forbes, T. W., Nolan, R. O., Schmidt, F. L., & Vanosdall, F. E. (1975). Driver performance measurement based on dynamic driver behavior patterns in rural, urban, suburban and freeway traffic. *Accid. Anal. Prev.*, 7, 257–280.

Gianutsos, R., & Beattie, A. (1992). Elemental driving simulator. In: Anonymous (Ed.), *Proceedings of the Johns Hopkins National Search for Computing Applications to Assist Persons with Disabilities* (pp. 117–120). Los Alamitos,CA: IEEE Computer Society Press.

Gianutsos, R. (1994). Driving advisement with the Elemental Driving Simulator (EDS): When less suffices. *Behav. Res. Meth. Instrum. Comput.*, 26(2), 183–186.

Gianutsos, R., & DeLibero, V. (1999). Reported driving, self-appraisal and simulator performance in younger and older drivers. In: Anonymous, *Transportation Research Board*.

Hunt, L. A., Murphy, C. F., Carr, D., Duchek, J. M., Buckles, V., & Morris, J. C. (1997). Reliability of the Washington University Road Test: A performance-based assessment for drivers with dementia of the Alzheimer type. *Arch. Neurol.*, 54(June), 707–712.

Janke, M. K., & Eberhard, J. (1998). Assessing medically impaired older drivers in a licensing agency setting. *Accid. Anal. Prev.*, 30(3), 347–361.

Klavora, P., Gaskovski, P., Martin, K., Forsyth, R. D., Heslegrave, R. J., Young, M., & Quinn, R. P. (1995). The effects of Dynavision rehabilitation on behind-the-wheel driving ability and selected psychomotor abilities of persons after stroke. *Am. J. Occup. Ther.*, 49(6), 534–542.

Lundqvist, A., & Ronnberg, J. (2001). Driving problems and adaptive driving behaviour after brain injury: A qualitative assessment. *Neuropsychol. Rehabil.*, 11(2), 171–185.

Malfetti, J. L., & Winter, D. J. (1991). *Concerned about and Older Driver? A Guide for Families and Friends*. Washington, DC: AAA Foundation for Traffic Safety.

Malfetti, J. L., & Winter, D. J. (1992). *Drivers 55 Plus Test Your Own Performance: A Self-Rating Form of Questions, Facts and Suggestions for Safe Driving*. Washington, DC: AAA Foundation for Traffic Safety.

Odenheimer, G. L., Beaudet, M., Jette, A. M., Albert, M. S., Grande, L., & Minaker, K. L. (1994). Performance-based driving evaluation of the elderly driver: Safety, reliability, and validity. *J. Gerontol. Med. Sci.*, 49(4), M153–M159.

Owsley, C., McGwin, G., & Ball, K. (1998). Vision impairment, eye disease, and injurious motor vehicle crashes in the elderly. *Ophthalmic Epidemiol.*, 5, 101–113.

Owsley, C., Stalvey, B., Wells, J., & Sloane, M. E. (1999). Older drivers and cataract: Driving habits and crash risk. *J. Gerontol. Biol. Med. Sci.*, 54, M203–211.

Pidikiti, R. D., & Novack, T. A. (1991). The disabled driver: An unmet challenge. *Arch. Phys. Med. Rehabil.*, 72(2), 109–111.

Pierce, S. (1996). A roadmap for driver rehabilitation. *Occupational Therapy Practice*, (Oct), 30–38.

Staplin, L., Lococo, K. H., Stewart, J., & Decina, L. E. (1999). Safe mobility for older people note-book. *National Highway Traffic Safety Administration*. DOT HS 808 853.
Tant, M. L. M. (2002). Visual performance in homonymous hemianopia: Assessment, training and driving. (http://www.ub.rug.nl/eldoc/dis/ppsw/m.l.m.tant/)
Wood, J. M., & Mallon, K. (2001). Comparison of driving performance of young and old drivers (with and without visual impairment) measured during in-traffic conditions. *Optom. Vis. Sci.*, *78*(5), 343–349.

4

HUMAN FACTOR
CONSIDERATIONS
IN MOTOR VEHICLE
COLLISIONS

PHILIP SCHATZ AND FRANK G. HILLARY

The current chapter aims to present basic descriptive and epidemiologic data characterizing motor vehicle collisions (MVCs) and the human and collision factors that influence their likelihood. In doing so, the vehicular, environmental, and human factors contributing to MVCs will be discussed and the remainder of this text will consider these factors within the context of clinical populations. Thus, this chapter provides base rate information regarding the multiple factors that contribute to MVCs in the general population as a precursor to understanding the assessment of driving ability in neurologically impaired populations.

THE IMPORTANCE OF DRIVING ASSESSMENT

Driving assessment in clinical samples should, ideally, guarantee that individuals who are capable of driving have the opportunity to do so, as well as to reduce the possibility of MVCs caused by people who experience difficulty operating a motor vehicle. The resultant injuries and fatalities associated with the use of motorized vehicles are a harsh reality for most industrialized countries. Nearly 132 million passenger vehicles are driven on America's roads and highways each year, resulting in approximately 5 million reported MVCs and

4 million documented emergency room visits (CDC, 1998). MVCs accounted for over 43,000 fatalities in 1998, or 16 per 100,000 people (CDC, 1998), which is comparable to previous years where 44,599 and 41,798 total MVC related fatalities were logged (1990 and 1995, respectively). MVCs are the most common cause of trauma in males (25%, lifetime prevalence) and second most common in females (13.8%, lifetime prevalence) (NHTSA, 1998) and it is estimated that over 1% of the American population is involved in a MVC each year (Blanchard & Hickling, 1997). MVCs are the second most common cause of death and the most common cause of traumatic brain injury (TBI) in the United States, resulting in 3–5 million head injuries a year (Kraus & McArthur, 1996), and a large percentage of the nation's injuries and fatalities.

Motor vehicle operation remains integral to independent living in the United States, as nearly one in two residents of the United States owns and operates a passenger vehicle (NHTSA, 1998). The ability to legally operate a motor vehicle after neurologic insult or disease is critical for social and vocational independence, necessitating the accurate assessment of driving competence in the neurologically impaired population.

HUMAN FACTORS AND MVCS

The majority of vehicle collisions can be attributed to driver behavior (as opposed to vehicle or roadway factors), which was found to be responsible for 37,081 fatalities and more than 2 million serious injuries (NHTSA, 1998). Thus, examining specific driver behaviors and their role in MVCs remains critical to safety advancement on America's highways. Although a variety of contributing factors have been addressed in the literature, the most reviewed include (1), perception and information processing, (2) distraction, (3) driver experience, and (4) demographic factors of the driver. Additionally, specific behaviors, such as seatbelt use and examining specific aspects of MVC (e.g., collision factors) can improve our ability to identify the primary contributing factors that result in collision.

THE ROLE OF PERCEPTION AND INFORMATION PROCESSING IN MVCS

Several chapters in this text are dedicated to examining clinical populations and the relevant literatures outlining the specific cognitive factors that are important for safe operation of motor vehicles. More generally, in healthy adults sensory and perceptual skills and information processing have been identified as critical components for safe driving. It has been estimated that drivers receive nearly 90% of their information through vision. Scanning, tracking, and figure-ground discrimination have all been demonstrated to be critical in attending and reacting to objects external to the vehicle (Simms, 1985). Separately, research on the role of disrupted attention specifically identified changes in auditory selective attention as contributing to increased motor vehicle accident rates (Kahneman et al., 1973). More recently examiners noted that a great majority of non-fatal MVCs in youthful drivers have been attributed to errors in attention, visual search, speed relative to conditions, hazard recognition, and emergency maneuvering (McKnight & McKnight, 2000). In sum, attention and perception have been recognized as two critical features across separate models describing information processing in driving. Simms model (1985) emphasizes a perceptual-information processing framework in driving and work by van Zomeren, et al. (1988) again emphasized attentional and perceptual components in their list of six general impairments that influence the ability to safely operate a motor vehicle. In fact, human error in attention, perception, and information processing has been estimated to cause 90–95% of all accidents (Simms, 1985). Issues regarding the importance of perceptual and attentional skills will be discussed throughout the remainder of this text and are critical to consider in clinical samples with deficits in these areas.

Other examiners have focused on the interaction between specific environmental factors and critical cognitive factors thought to predict driver behavior. Environmental factors, such as road type, traffic conditions, and weather conditions, have different demand characteristics for the driver. These environmental factors likely influence scanning, attention and concentration, and information processing demands (Galski et al., 1998). Even simple vehicle characteristics, such as color have been shown to influence rate of MVC, with lighter-colored vehicles such as white or yellow significantly less likely to be involved in a passive MVC, which is described as a collision where the operator was not at fault (Lardelli-Claret et al., 2002). Other extra-vehicle environmental demands such as reversed-side driving conditions in foreign countries have been found to contribute to increased accident involvement, especially while traveling for pleasure on vacation (Petridou et al., 1997).

THE ROLE OF DISTRACTION IN MVCs

Other researchers have focused on within-vehicle distractions that may influence driving ability. For example, researchers have emphasized the importance of "temporary distraction" while driving as factors that may reduce driver effectiveness (Petridou & Moustaki, 2000). In one study, cigarette smoking was found to have a 150% increased risk for MVCs and smoking while driving was associated with higher risk of MVCs (Brison, 1990). Even so, other investigators have found that within-vehicle distractions as a contributory factor account for only about 2% of all fatal accidents (Stevens & Minton, 2001).

A more recent and controversial in-vehicle distraction that has received much attention over the past few years is the use of mobile phones while operating a motor vehicle. Use of mobile phones in motor vehicles is increasing and has been linked to decreased attention, especially for those over age 50, or when the conversation intensity increases (McKnight & McKnight, 1993). A widely recognized study examining mobile phone use found that use of mobile phones while driving increased the likelihood of collisions by 400%, and "hand's free" mobile phones offered no appreciable safety advantage (Redelmeier & Tibshirani, 1997). These findings have come under some scrutiny (Maclure & Mittleman, 1997) and more recent investigations have revealed mild to moderate increases in MVCs in mobile phone users. For example, one study surveying drivers showed an increase of 38% in MVCs in mobile phone users (Laberge-Nadeau et al., 2003). Other examiners have noted that performance of the driver is most dramatically affected in the areas of reaction time, mental load, and vehicular control during mobile phone use (Lamble et al., 1999; Consiglio et al., 2003; Hancock et al., 2003). While it appears that mobile phone use may increase the likelihood of MVC, an important issue to be addressed is the specific reason for this increased probability. This has been difficult to ascertain. It has been emphasized that, in Japan, MVCs may be most likely to occur while the phone operator was dialing the to-be-called phone number but that in the United States a majority of the MVCs occur during conversations (NHTSA, 1998). Examiners finding support for the former have noted that mobile phone usage in motor vehicles with "hands-free" systems may not be necessarily safer unless dialing is voice activated (Consiglio et al., 2003).

Much of the driving experience is highly automated and when circumstances are not overly demanding, drivers have historically occupied themselves with other activities while driving. For example, examiners have noted that taking on the phone while operating a vehicle may be no worse than any other within-vehicle activity that divides the driver's attention including, eating, drinking, conversing, and listening to the radio. Separately, examiners have cautioned lawmakers against widespread legislation against mobile phone use in motor vehicles due to the additional communicative advantages provided drivers in emergency situations (Consiglio et al., 2003). In sum, the issue regarding mobile phone use during motor vehicle operation is complicated and, ultimately, will require legal mandates that circumscribe their use.

DRIVER EXPERIENCE AND MVC LIKELIHOOD

Not surprisingly, examiners have noted that more experienced drivers are generally better drivers and are less likely to be involved in MVCs (Maycock et al., 1991). The reasons for the improved driving capacity in experienced drivers is related to several factors including improved automaticity and an advanced or mature perception of driving scenarios. For example, (Renge, 2000) found that more experienced drivers performed better than novices in understanding other road users' communicative signals and, in an investigation of training road hazard perception, Crick & McKenna (1991) noted that experience influences the ability to quickly detect road hazards. More experienced drivers may outperform their novice counterparts by creating a superior "mental model" of driving situations. Such mental models provide the driver with a schema to predict the likelihood of safety (Vogel et al., 2003).

DEMOGRAPHICS FACTORS AND MVC

An important human factor to consider when examining MVCs is the influence of a specific demographic or cohort on collision probability. One such factor is age. It is now well established that teenagers and young adults are more likely to be involved in motor vehicle collisions and a second sample with increased likelihood to be involved in MVCs is the elderly (Zhang et al., 1998). This bimodal distribution accounts for an appreciable portion of the MVCs each year. For example, older adults have one of the highest crash rates per mile traveled compared to most other groups (Williams & Carsten, 1989), even considering the fact that they drive fewer miles, make fewer trips, and drive less in demanding driving situations (e.g., night time, during rush hour) (Lyman et al., 2001). The reasons for increased MVCs in older adults have been attributed to medical conditions, improper rule following, and difficulty at intersections (Lyman et al., 2001). These factors are important to consider given that the most common method for travel for elderly people is driving an automobile (USDOT, 1998).

In younger adults, the rate of MVC has been noted to decrease significantly from age 16 to age 19. Researchers have shown that the incidence of serious collisions decline as early as 6 months after licensure (Williams & Carsten, 1989; Mayhew et al., 2003). This dramatic drop-off over just a few years likely indicates an important interaction between maturity and increasing driving experience. When examining the predictors of teenage MVCs, examiners have noted that the two most important factors determining higher likelihood are use of alcohol (Williams et al., 1986) and presence of other teenagers in the car (Chen et al., 2000). Similarly, Zhang et al. (1998) found that younger drivers were at higher risks for alcohol related MVC, collisions during nights and weekends, single vehicle collisions and collisions resulting from performing overtaking maneuvers.

USE OF SEATBELTS AND THEIR INFLUENCE ON INJURY IN MVCs

The national incidence for seatbelt usage is rising (70%) (NHTSA, 2001), yet it remains imperative that health care professionals emphasize the use of safety restraints to their patients. Seatbelts have been scrutinized under all types of collision configurations and remain the most consistent preventative mechanism against injury. For example, it has been estimated that during the 1996 calendar year, seatbelt use may have saved 10,414 lives, and 90,425 lives cumulatively since 1975 (NHTSA, 1998). Furthermore, in cases where brain injuries are sustained during MVCs, the use of seatbelts has been associated with less injury severity (Hillary et al., 2001; Hillary et al., 2002). Taken together, these studies indicate that using a seatbelt not only prevents fatality and injury from occurring during MVC, but may also reduce the severity of injuries when they do occur.

While a variety of factors seem to be associated with seatbelt use, interestingly, one determining factor influencing the use of a seatbelt by the driver is the

TABLE 4.1　Percentage of Patients Wearing a Seatbelt
at the Time of Injury by Demographic Characteristics.

Age	< 25	45%
	25–60	52%
	>60	68%
Sex	Male	45%
	Female	63%
Race	Caucasians	56%
	African	34%
	Americans	40%
	Others	
Income	<$20,000	33%
	>$20,000	55%
Position in vehicle	Driver	57%
	Passenger	43%

use of a seatbelt by someone else in the vehicle. Hong et al. (1998) found that when the front seat passenger uses a seatbelt, the driver was 77% likely to also be wearing a seatbelt and this frequency of safety restraint use dropped to only 44% when the front seat passenger was without a seatbelt. Wilson (1990) showed that non-use of a safety belt were higher sensation seekers, more impulsive, and accumulated more traffic violations than those who used safety restraints. These factors will be critical to consider in clinical samples that may have a history of sensation seeking or impulsivity (e.g., TBI). Lerner et al. (2001) noted a significant difference in the influence of gender, socioeconomic status, and law enforcement (e.g., primary versus secondary seatbelt use enforcement) on seatbelt use. In this study, 45% of the men and 63% of the women used a seatbelt. Table 4.1 provides a breakdown of the different demographic variables and their influence on seatbelt usage in injured motor vehicle occupants.

COLLISION FACTORS

Analyses of specific collision configurations have provided investigators with critical information about the relationship between specific driving characteristics, collision types, and occupant injury. One method for examining collision factors has been through the use of the Fatality Accident Reporting System (FARS), a national database established in 1975 providing researchers with the ability to analyze the basic collision configurations associated with higher probability of occupant fatality. For example, operators of small vehicles are much less likely to be involved in collisions, operators of smaller/lighter vehicles are more likely to be injured in two-car collisions (Evans & Frick, 1993). One explanation for this dissociation is that drivers of smaller vehicles adjust their driving behavior due to their increased risk for injury in collisions, thus reducing involvement in MVCs.

An important question to consider is whether or not individuals with neurological impairment continue to implicitly calculate such subtle factors when operating a motor vehicle. This is particularly important in individuals who may have deficits in judgment and/or inhibition, and, therefore, no longer adjust their style of driving.

Other interactions between specific collision variables and driver behavior that often result in severe injury should be considered when providing consultation to patients before they resume driving. For example, investigations of real-world collisions have revealed that lateral impact collisions (i.e., where the vehicle is struck from the side) and frontal collisions with a fixed structure (i.e., where the vehicle strikes a building, or unyielding object such as a utility pole) result in the most severe brain injuries when examining a brain injured sample (Hillary et al., 2002). In this study, lateral collisions most often occurred at intersections within major metropolitan areas, and these findings are important to consider when working with elderly drivers because they are significantly more likely than younger adults to be involved in collisions at intersections (Keskinen et al., 1998). It may be helpful for clinicians to address certain driving behaviors with patients before and after driving resumption.

STATE REQUIREMENTS FOR REPORTING NEUROLOGICALLY IMPAIRED DRIVERS

Following neurological insult, neither the privilege of driving nor the assessment of driving ability is federally mandated in the United States. As such, the laws requiring the assessment of driving ability following diagnosis varies from state to state. As recently as the late 1980s, physicians allowed their patient to make the final decision whether or not to continue driving, perhaps motivated by a respect for the individual and a desire to promote patient autonomy (Reuben et al., 1988). By 1990, only 15 states authorized physicians to report impaired drivers and only 7 states mandated such reporting (Pidikiti & Novack, 1991). At present, there remains a lack of commonality in driving assessment laws among the states, which contributes to the variation in reporting laws from state to state. In some states (e.g., New Jersey), if individuals have a condition affecting their mental or physical ability to operate a motor vehicle, they are obligated to notify to Department of Motor Vehicles (DMV). However, in New York, for example, individuals with a neurological condition maintain a valid license until the time of renewal, when they are required to report any changes in their mental and physical status since their last application (Gianutsos, 1989). In addition, the reporting requirements across states may be specific to the disorder being reported (e.g., Delaware, New Jersey, and Nevada require reporting for epilepsy; California, for dementia). Furthermore, the majority of states either do not permit health care providers to report impairments that may compromise driving (Haselkorn et al., 1998) or merely allow physicians to report patients on a permissive basis (Malinowski & Petrucelli, 1997).

In the United Kingdom drivers are required to inform the Driver and Vehicle Licensing Agency (DVLA) if they have any disability which is likely to last for more than 3 months and which may affect their fitness to drive (Hawley, 2001). Taking a similar stance in the United States, the American Medical Association stated that it is "desirable and ethical" for physicians to notify their respective DMV if an impaired patient under their treatment fails to restrict his or her driving appropriately (AMA, 1999). Despite this documented mandate, there has been little carry-over to standardized practice.

Physicians do recognize driving safety as an important public health issue; 77% reported discussing driving issues with potentially unsafe drivers and 14% reported their patients to the DMV (Drickamer & Marottoli, 1993). However, many physicians are not well informed regarding state reporting laws (King et al., 1992) and may not be familiar with the reporting process. For example, in one investigation more than 28% of all geriatricians did not know how to report patients with dementia who were potentially dangerous drivers (Cable et al., 2000). In the absence of standardized reporting procedures, physicians' self-reported practices often go against practicality or their own patients' wishes. For example, studies have indicated that 86% of providers reported that they would contact state authorities despite objections from their patient, and 73% would contact authorities despite objections from the patient's family.

This lack of standardization also impacts service delivery. For example, one study found that despite the prevalence of TBI, few drivers reported receiving formal advice about driving after their injury (Hawley, 2001), save for advice from family members or non-physician health care professionals. In one survey, nearly 63% of individuals who had sustained head injury had not been professionally evaluated for competency (Fisk et al., 1998). Researchers have noted the importance of diagnosing driving ability with standardized, psychometrically sound instruments, rather than clinical judgment (Lambert & Engum, 1992), however, establishing a single nationally recognized protocol has proven difficult. As evidenced throughout this text, there exists a wide body of research on the strengths and weaknesses of tests of basic attention and concentration, neuropsychological test batteries, driving simulators, and on-road assessments in the prediction of driving ability.

CONCLUSION

Taken together, literature from varied sources reveals a variety of scenarios where driving ability may be influenced in healthy adults. These same motor vehicle and driver behavior factors have the potential to differentially influence driving ability in a neurologically impaired population and require consideration when assessing the driving privileges of patients. The driving candidate's motor and cognitive abilities (e.g., attention, concentration, impulsivity, and insight) are typically the focus of assessment, however, other factors such as internal (e.g., mobile phone use and presence of passengers) and external environmental factors (e.g., roadway type, level of traffic, and day versus night driving) also require consideration.

REFERENCES

AMA. (1999). American Medical Association: Opinions of Council on Ethical and Judicial Affairs Opinion.

Blanchard, E. B., & Hickling, E. J. (1997). *After the Crash: Assessment and Treatment of Motor Vehicle Accident Survivors*. Washington, DC: American Psychological Association.

Brison, R. J. (1990). Risk of automobile accidents in cigarette smokers. *Can. J. Public Health, 81*(2), 102–106.

Cable, G., Reisner, M., Gerges, S., & Thirumavalavan, V. (2000). Knowledge, attitudes, and practices of geriatricians regarding patients with dementia who are potentially dangerous automobile drivers: A national survey. *J. Am. Geriatr. Soc., 48*(1), 14–17.

Center for Disease Control (1998). *National Vital Statistics Report* (Vol. 48).

Chen, L. H., Baker, S. P., Braver, E. R., & Li, G. (2000). Carrying passengers as a risk factor for crashes fatal to 16- and 17-year-old drivers. *JAMA, 283*(12), 1578–1582.

Consiglio, W., Driscoll, P., Witte, M., & Berg, W. P. (2003). Effect of cellular telephone conversations and other potential interference on reaction time in a braking response. *Accid. Anal. Prev., 35*(4), 495–500.

Crick, J., & McKenna, F. P. (1991). Hazard perception: Can it be trained? *Proceedings of Manchester University Seminar: Behavioural Research in Road Safety II*. Manchester England: Manchester University.

Drickamer, M. A., & Marottoli, R. A. (1993). Physician responsibility in driver assessment. *Am. J. Med. Sci., 306*(5), 277–281.

Evans, L., & Frick, M. C. (1993). Mass ratio and relative driver fatality risk in two-vehicle crashes. *Accid. Anal. Prev., 25*(2), 213–224.

Fisk, G. D., Schneider, J. J., & Novack, T. A. (1998). Driving following traumatic brain injury: Prevalence, exposure, advice and evaluations. *Brain Injury, 12*(8), 683–695.

Galski, T., Ehle, H. T., & Willimas, B. (1998). Estimates of driving abilities and skills in different conditions. *Am. J. Occup. Ther., 52*(4), 268–274.

Gianutsos, R. (1989). A word to survivors of brain injury who would resume driving and their families. *NYS Head Injury Assoc. Newslett., 9*(1).

Hancock, P. A., Lesch, M., & Simmons, L. (2003). The distraction effects of phone use during a crucial driving maneuver. *Accid. Anal. Prev., 35*(4), 501–514.

Haselkorn, J. K., Mueller, B. A., & Rivara, F. A. (1998). Characteristics of drivers and driving record after traumatic and nontraumatic brain injury. *Arch. Phys. Med. Rehab., 79*(7), 738–742.

Hawley, C. A. (2001). Return to driving after head injury. *J. Neurol. Neurosurg. Psychiatry, 70*(6), 761–766.

Hillary, F., Moelter, S. T., Schatz, P., & Chute, D. L. (2001). Seatbelts contribute to location of lesion in moderate to severe closed head trauma. *Arch. Clin. Neuropsychol., 16*(2), 171–181.

Hillary, F. G., Schatz, P., Moelter, S. T., Lowry, J. B., Ricker, J. H., & Chute, D. L. (2002). Motor vehicle collision factors influence severity and type of TBI. *Brain Inj., 16*(8), 729–741.

Hong, S., Kim, D., Kritkausky, K., & Rashid, R. (1998). Effects of imitative behaviour on seat belt usage: Three field observational studies. Paper presented at the *Proceedings of the 42nd Annual Meeting of the Human Factors and Ergonomics Society*.

Kahneman, D., Ben-Ishai, R., & Lotan, M. (1973). Relation of a test of attention to road accidents. *J. Appl. Psychol., 58*(1), 113–115.

Keskinen, E., Ota, H., & Katila, A. (1998). Older drivers fail in intersections: Speed discrepancies between older and younger male drivers. *Accid. Anal. Prev., 30*(3), 323–330.

King, D., Benbow, S. J., & Barrett, J. A. (1992). The law and medical fitness to drive – A study of doctors' knowledge. *Postgrad. Med. J.*, *68*(802), 624–628.

Kraus, J. F., & McArthur, D. L. (1996). Epidemiologic aspects of brain injury. *Neurol. Clin.*, *14*(2), 435–450.

Laberge-Nadeau, C., Maag, U., Bellavance, F., Lapierre, S. D., Desjardins, D., Messier, S. et al. (2003). Wireless telephones and the risk of road crashes. *Accid. Anal. Prev.*, *35*(5), 649–660.

Lambert, E. W., & Engum, E. (1992). Construct validity of the cognitive behavioral driver's inventory: Age, diagnosis and driving ability. *J. Cogn. Rehab.*, *10*(3), 32–45.

Lamble, D., Kauranen, T., Laakso, M., & Summala, H. (1999). Cognitive load and detection thresholds in car following situations: Safety implications for using mobile (cellular) telephones while driving. *Accid. Anal. Prev.*, *31*(6), 617–623.

Lardelli-Claret, P., De Dios Luna-Del-Castillo, J., Juan Jimenez-Moleon, J., Femia-Marzo, P., Moreno-Abril, O., & Bueno-Cavanillas, A. (2002). Does vehicle color influence the risk of being passively involved in a collision? *Epidemiology*, *13*(6), 721–724.

Lerner, E. B., Jehle, D. V., Billittier, A. J. IV., Moscati, R. M., Connery, C. M., & Stiller, G. (2001). The influence of demographic factors on seatbelt use by adults injured in motor vehicle crashes. *Accid. Anal. Prev.*, *33*(5), 659–662.

Lyman, J. M., McGwin, G. Jr., & Sims, R. V. (2001). Factors related to driving difficulty and habits in older drivers. *Accid. Anal. Prev.*, *33*(3), 413–421.

Maclure, M., & Mittleman, M. A. (1997). Cautions about car telephones and collisions. *N. Engl. J. Med.*, *336*(7), 501–502.

Malinowski, M., & Petrucelli, E. (1997). *Update of medical review practices and procedures in U.S. and Canadian Driver Licensing Programs*. Washington, DC: Federal Highway Administration.

Maycock, G., Lockwood, C. R., & Lester, J. (1991). *The accident liability of car drivers. TRL Research Report RR315*. Crowthome: Transport Research Laboratory.

Mayhew, D. R., Simpson, H. M., & Pak, A. (2003). Changes in collision rates among novice drivers during the first months of driving. *Accid. Anal. Prev.*, *35*(5), 683–691.

McKnight, A. J., & McKnight, A. S. (1993). The effect of cellular phone use upon driver attention. *Accid. Anal. Prev.*, *25*(3), 259–265.

McKnight, A. J., & McKnight, A. S. (2000). The behavioral contributors to highway crashes of youthful drivers. *Annu. Proc. Assoc. Adv. Automot. Med.*, *44*, 321–333.

NHTSA (1998). *National Center for Statistics and Analysis: Traffic Safety Facts 1998, DOT HS 808 983*. Washington, DC: US Department of Transportation.

NHTSA (2001). *National Highway Traffic Safety Association: Status of Occupant Protection in America*U.S. Department of Transportation.

Petridou, E., & Moustaki, M. (2000). Human factors in the causation of road traffic crashes. *Eur. J. Epidemiol.*, *16*(9), 819–826.

Petridou, E., Askitopoulou, H., Vourvahakis, D., Skalkidis, Y., & Trichopoulos, D. (1997). Epidemiology of road traffic accidents during pleasure traveling: The evidence from the island of Crete. *Accid. Anal. & Prev.*, *29*(5), 687–693.

Pidikiti, R. D., & Novack, T. A. (1991). The disabled driver: An unmet challenge. *Arch. Phys. Med. Rehab.*, *72*(2), 109–111.

Redelmeier, D. A., & Tibshirani, R. J. (1997). Association between cellular-telephone calls and motor vehicle collisions. *N. Engl. J. Med.*, *336*(7), 453–458.

Renge, K. (2000). Effect of experience on drivers' decoding process of roadway interpersonal communications. *Ergonomics*, *43*(1), 27–39.

Reuben, D. B., Silliman, R. A., & Traines, M. (1988). The aging driver. Medicine, policy, and ethics. *J. Am. Geriatr. Soc.*, *36*(12), 1135–1142.

Simms, B. (1985). The assessment of the disabled for driving: A preliminary report. *Int. Rehab. Med.*, *7*(4), 187–192.

Stevens, A., & Minton, R. (2001). In-vehicle distraction and fatal accidents in England and Wales. *Accid. Anal. Prev.*, *33*(4), 539–545.

USDOT (1998). *Highway Statistics Summary, 1995–1998*. Washington, DC: Federal Highway Administration.

van Zomeren, A. H., Brouwer, W. H., Rothengatter, J. A., & Snoek, J. W. (1988). Fitness to drive a car after recovery from severe head injury. *Arch. Phys. Med. Rehab.*, *69*(2), 90–96.

Vogel, K., Kircher, A., Alm, H., & Nilsson, L. (2003). Traffic sense – which factors influence the skill to predict the development of traffic scenes? *Accid. Anal. Prev.*, *35*(5), 749–762.

Williams, A. F., & Carsten, O. (1989). Driver age and crash involvement. *Am. J. Public Health*, *79*(3), 326–327.

Williams, A. F., Lund, A. K., & Preusser, D. F. (1986). Drinking and driving among high school students. *Int. J. Addict.*, *21*(6), 643–655.

Wilson, R. J. (1990). The relationship between seat belt non-use to personality, lifestyle and driving record. *Health Education Research: Theory and Practice*, *5*(2), 175–185.

Zhang, J., Fraser, S., Lindsay, J., Clarke, K., & Mao, Y. (1998). Age-specific patterns of factors related to fatal motor vehicle traffic crashes: Focus on young and elderly drivers. *Public Health*, *112*(5), 289–295.

5

DRIVING AND TRAUMATIC BRAIN INJURY

C. ALAN HOPEWELL

Traumatic brain injury (TBI) is defined as brain damage secondary to an externally inflicted trauma. It is an ongoing "silent epidemic" with an annual incidence of approximately 1.4 million cases per year in the United States (Center for Disease Control, 2006). Conservative estimates are that approximately 500,000 require hospitalization and 80,000 suffer from chronic disability of some kind. TBI is the leading cause of death and disability in people younger than 45 years of age, with an overall mortality rate of 25 deaths per 100,000. An estimated 5.3 million Americans, a little more than 2% of the US population, currently live with disabilities from TBI, according to a 2006 report by the Centers for Disease Control and Prevention. Other statistics reported by the CDC indicate that each year, one million people are treated and released in hospital emergency rooms, and 50,000 people die. The age of peak incidence of head injury is 15–24 years, although the distribution is bimodal with geriatrics being the next frequently injured. The risk of TBI in men is twice the risk in women, and the risk is higher in adolescents, young adults, and people older than 75 years – exactly those most likely to be involved in motor vehicle accidents. While those who are very seriously injured may readily be identified as being precluded from future motor vehicle operations, approximately three-quarters are diagnosed as having suffered a mild-to-moderate injury – injuries that can be subtle, persistent, and which may present potentially long-term disability. One such disability is the potential risk for preclusion of driving.

One of the most challenging aspects for the TBI survivor is that many times such individuals suffer little outward physical manifestation of injury. As a result, some of the long-term sequelae resulting from TBI may not be readily addressed, this includes physical, cognitive, psychological, and social impairments. Not surprising issues of driving may not be considered until later, or may not be considered at all.

The pathophysiology of TBI can be considered at various levels, including injury resulting from the direct mechanical impact of the trauma and at the neuronal level of the brain's response to the trauma. Falls and motor vehicle accidents are the leading cause of TBI (CDC, 2006) with both resulting in a combination of primary and secondary injuries. These can include tearing and bruising of the brain as a result of impact with inner surfaces of the brain and injuries resulting from the momentum of the brain's impact against a skull that has been decelerated, or may often occur in blunt force trauma. These injuries commonly result in edema within a cranial vault which does not expand, resulting in secondary compression that can have profound long-term effects. The primary injuries caused by direct mechanical impact of trauma may be either "focal" or "diffuse." Focal injuries include contusion, intracerebral hematoma, intracranial hemorrhage, or focal hypoxic-ischemic injury. Contusion is the most common focal injury and is the result of acceleration–deceleration forces and the angular and transitional movements of the head, causing the brain to impact on the bony protuberances of the skull producing coupe (at the site of impact) and contrecoupe (away from the site of impact) injury. Among the diffuse injuries, diffuse axonal shearing is the most common and is caused by angular or rotational acceleration of the head producing shearing and tearing of the axons. Brain edema and swelling, hypoxic brain damage, and vascular injury comprise other types of diffuse brain injuries. Post-concussion syndrome can also result from TBI and can present with headaches, spasticity, dizziness, reduced coordination, sensory dysfunction, memory losses, problems in concentrating, difficulty in perceiving, sequencing, judgment and communication, fatigue, emotional volatility.

The results of these injuries include long-term sensory, cognitive, and motor deficits which can impair vehicle operation. Despite this, many survivors may not receive formal consultation, advice, or treatment to help return them safely to driving or to determine those who are at high risk for such return (Fisk et al., 1998). To understand driving better following TBI, a survey of driving status, driving exposure, advice received about driving and evaluations of driving competency was administered to 83 TBI survivors by Fisk et al. (1998). The majority of survey participants had experienced either moderate or severe TBI based on the Glasgow Coma Scale, and 60% had reported that they were currently active drivers. These survivors reportedly had received advice about driving from family members, physicians or non-physician health care professionals, but over half (63%) had not been professionally evaluated for driving competency. Results from the study also suggested that cognitive, sensory, or motor deficits after injury may negatively affect driving skills, and the authors also felt that the presence of high-driving exposure coupled with a lack of widespread driving fitness testing, suggested that some TBI survivors have characteristics that may elevate their risk for vehicle crashes.

Nonetheless, current research indicates that 32–85% of individuals who sustain a TBI return to driving (Fisk et al., 1998; Hawley, 2001; Coleman et al., 2002; Schultheis et al., 2002; Formisano et al., 2005; Pietrapiana et al., 2005; Rapport et al., 2006). This is despite the fact that such individuals may be at increased risk of engaging in unsafe driving behavior (Fisk et al., 1998; Hawley, 2001; Coleman et al., 2002; Formisano et al., 2005; Pietrapiana et al., 2005). The high percentage of individuals returning to driving is not surprising given the fact that cessation of driving has been related to difficulties with employment (Devaney-Serio & Devens, 1994), depression (Marottoli et al., 1997), poor social integration, and the inability to engage in activities outside of the home (Dawson & Chipman, 1995).

DRIVING ISSUES

The decrease in independence which is frequently encountered after TBI can create new problems for individuals, their families, and rehabilitation agencies. It is true that the increased emphasis on rehabilitation in recent years has made it possible for large numbers of neuropsychologically impaired individuals to return to some level of community functioning. However, the rehabilitation of potential motor vehicle operators is not to be treated in the same fashion as the routine physical therapy of the same disabled individuals. Returning a cognitively impaired individual to motor vehicle operation is not the same as helping him or her to walk. This situation results in increased responsibility not only among TBI survivors wishing to return to driving, but also among rehabilitation professionals working with these issues. This may also well contribute to a therapist–patient relationship in which there is a special relationship requiring a duty to protect or warn where high risk is suspected or determined (Pettis, 1992).

With recent advances in medicine and rehabilitation, increasing numbers of brain injury survivors have led to a dramatic expansion in the number of individuals who may return to motor vehicle operations after injury or illness. The passage of the Americans with Disabilities Act (ADA) encourages individuals with both physical as well as mental (cognitive) disabilities to seek greater community access, including access to motor vehicles. Other than questions relating to mental competency in general, it is hard to imagine questions of a more practical, applied, or important nature than those questions related to fitness to operate a motor vehicle.

At the same time, all American legal jurisdictions, as well as those of most other developed countries, place substantial restrictions upon the ability of some individuals with disabilities to procure or to maintain an unrestricted driver's license. The result is that two strongly competing interests are at stake when a legal jurisdiction imposes driving limitations. First of all, such restrictions reflect the need of the State to protect the public from the consequences and acts of persons who are incompetent to drive or who demonstrate an unacceptable level of driving risk, as well as the need to protect such persons from themselves. On the other hand, driving in a developed society has become the predominant means toward independence, the ability to earn a living, and the fulfillment of a significant number of personal goals. The freedom to work, to travel, to shop, and to seek recreational outlets contributes significantly to our independence.

MEDICAL AND "DRIVING SKILL" MODELS ARE NECESSARY, BUT NOT SUFFICIENT

Two models which have most frequently been applied to the rehabilitation of the impaired driver are the "medical model" and the "driving skills" model.

Medical model

- A "pathological condition," "disease," or "disability" exists; (viz., "brain injury");
- Such a condition may be "diagnosed;"
- "Treatments" or a "cure" are available, often of a medication or physical intervention nature;
- Such treatments need to be directed, supervised, or prescribed by medical personnel;
- Response to treatment results in "cure" or improvement.

Driving skills model

- The successful operation of a motor vehicle is a learned and expressed behavioral skill;
- Knowledge of driving laws and regulations is a critical component of risk reduction;
- Inexperienced or poor drivers lack skills which may be learned in an educational environment;
- Educators, teachers, or regulatory personnel such as Department of Public Safety Officers may provide instruction or evaluation of "driving skills;"
- Such skills are maintained and strengthened by practice.

In considering the possible resumption of driving after TBI, elements of both of these models are necessary, but they cannot be considered to be sufficient to address the task at hand, either singularly or in combination. The *medical model*, while addressing medical and some rehabilitation issues, fails to recognize the functional and dynamic nature of driving as a functional behavior, and fails to consider critical psychological factors. The model also relies heavily on the medicalization of the rehabilitation process and the use of medical personnel to the relative exclusion of non-medical teachers, supervisors, and rehabilitation experts. The *driving skill* model likewise fails to account for psychological factors, to include psychiatric, executive, and information processing models. The model may also neglect critical medical issues (e.g., Does the TBI survivor demonstrate well preserved driving skills on a state driving examination yet suffer from a seizure disorder?). The model may also neglect developmental issues, such as disproportionate risk issues with teen and aged drivers; risk which may be considerably exacerbated by brain injury. And finally, neither model adequately delineates risk identification, risk management, or risk/benefit decision strategies.

The operation of a motor vehicle is, after all, a functional behavior (or rather, a complete repertoire of behaviors). As such, the inability to drive a car is not a medical disease to be diagnosed or treated but is rather a set of greatly impaired functional behaviors that may be evaluated and modified. Although medical conditions undoubtedly affect driving abilities and physicians should be part of the overall decision-making process, the evaluation and prediction of complex behavior must remain within the realm of the psychological, rather than the medical model.

Likewise, driving skill models make use of the reasonable and yet erroneous idea that numerous psychomotor abilities, such as visual scanning, attention, overall driving knowledge (e.g., how to shift gears, etc.), and reaction time, interact to form a hypothetical construct of driving skill, and that the more "driving skill" one has, the better a driver one will be. This popular notion, combined with the idea that knowledge of traffic laws is important, has been the basis for all state licensing examinations. In reality, these examinations, whether written, in vivo, or both, are actually among the *least* predictive of actual driving behavior or accident risk (Wallace & Crancer, 1971). A substantial body of research in this area has demonstrated that knowledge of driving regulations as well as basic psychomotor abilities, such as coordination and reaction time, are among the *least* predictive factors of accident risk (McFarland et al., 1954).

The realization that motor vehicle operation requires an extremely complex repertoire of interacting behaviors among emotional regulation, information processing, and motor response components has led authors to propose more sophisticated models to predict driving behavior. For example, an early study based on a perceptual information processing model (Mihal & Barrett, 1976) confirmed that such a model could be successfully used to document stable differences in information processing.

NEUROPSYCHOLOGICAL MODELS

If psychomotor abilities and knowledge of traffic laws are of relatively little importance in the eventual prediction of driving risk, what factors are important? A review of the scientific literature suggests that five major personality factors account for most of the variance in driving risk (Greenshields & Platt, 1967; Schuster, 1968; Selzer et al., 1968; Harano et al., 1975; Garretson & Peck, 1982; Miller & Schuster, 1983; Peck & Kuan, 1983; Noyes, 1985; Tsuang et al., 1985; Cremona, 1986). Cremona's article in particular reports research estimating that 90% of all automobile accidents are caused by human error and that over 25% of these accidents were related to psychiatric factors, including alcohol. An investigation of fatal accidents by Selzer et al. (1968) indicated that 20% of fatalities investigated were found to have been acutely upset by an event that had occurred during the 6-hour period immediately preceding the fatal accident. Such findings have obvious implications for TBI survivors experiencing symptoms such as episodic dyscontrol, explosive disorder, attentional lapses, information processing disturbances, depression, and a variety of other cognitive and affective symptoms.

Psychological factors contributing to accident risk, in descending order of importance (as determined from literature review), are as follows: (1) previous driving and accident/violation history, adjusted for exposure; (2) general personality and attitudinal factors; (3) pattern and severity of alcohol/substance abuse; (4) nature and extent of psychiatric disturbance; and (5) basic psychomotor abilities, assuming no disqualifying conditions, such as blindness, exist. All of these may also be considerably disturbed or worsened in conjunction with brain injury.

In addition, when dealing with issues presented by the individual with TBI, cognitive factors must be considered as these functions are often disrupted by injury, and can be most critical for driving. The paradox is that while the operation of a motor vehicle requires adequate basic psychomotor competence for over-learned tasks, traffic participation simultaneously demands a great deal of flexibility and executive processing in order to cope with even routine traffic situations.

It has been suggested that cognitive problems are highlighted when task demands exceed capacity and when one or more areas of functioning are required simultaneously, such as in driving. Consistent with this idea, some researchers have indicated that individuals with brain injury drive slower to compensate for their delayed reaction time (Stokx & Gaillard, 1986). Similarly, vulnerabilities in divided attention may be more apparent in novel situations or during times of high-traffic density when older drivers may be overwhelmed (Parasuraman & Nestor, 1993; Lengenfelder et al., 2002).

However, some aspects of cognition, such as procedural memory are frequently spared after TBI, and as such some aspects of driving can be well preserved (Brouwer et al., 2002). Galski et al. (1993) differentiate between what an individual does to operate a vehicle (e.g., press pedals, turn steering wheel) versus "how the person drives the vehicle," thereby suggesting that execution of these over-learned skills may be problematic even if the memory for the procedure is intact (p. 394). In general these procedural or rote aspects of driving are believed to represent the most basic of skills necessary for successful driving (Michon, 1985). Given the constant variability in driving demands when an individual is on the road (e.g., changes in environment, unexpected events), it is not surprising that higher demands (strategic and tactical) can impact the execution of the more basic behaviors.

Interest has therefore increasingly turned to investigation of multifunctional information processing tasks which are now felt to be among the best overall predictors of complex tasks such as driving (Heaton & Pendleton, 1981). Early on, Heaton and Pendleton hypothesized that tests such as Trail Making and Categories would predict complex behaviors such as driving because they tap functions of decision-making, mental flexibility, analysis and organization of novel material, abstraction, problem solving, and complex visuomotor responding. These authors assumed that moderately or severely depressed scores on a number of these types of neuropsychological tests might serve as predictors for the disqualification of the disabled driver.

Such assumptions subsequently began to be supported by independent work done at Louisiana Tech University, where tests such as Trail Making (B), Digit Symbol, and the Driver Performance Test were found to be among the best predictors of automobile driving among brain-injured drivers (Hale, 1986–1987). Other measures, such as the Symbol Digit Modalities test (Gouvier et al., 1989) and the Cognitive Behavioral Driver's Inventory (Engum et al., 1988b), have also been found to be useful in discriminating competent from incompetent drivers.

Current research strongly emphasizes investigation of the executive functions which are critical for driving, and which include mental flexibility, information processing, multi-tasking, tactical and strategic decision-making, and impulse control. In sum many areas of cognitive functioning have been implicated with regard to driving difficulties in this population. The following five cognitive domains are consistently addressed in the literature: attention/concentration, processing speed, visual memory, visual–spatial skills, and executive functioning.

In addition, co-morbid psychiatric conditions are known to increase accident risk, and such conditions are often noted before, after, and concomitant with TBI. In their review of the psychiatric sequelae of TBI, for example, Rao and Lyketsos (2002) found the following incidence of co-morbid psychiatric impairment in survivors:

Disorders	Percentage incidence (%)
Major depression	6–77
Mania	3–9
Anxiety	11–70
Apathy	10
Psychosis	2–20
Behavioral dyscontrol (major and minor variant)	11–100

Such figures are consistent with the co-morbid patterns reported by Jackson et al. (1992). The Jackson et al., study found through an orthogonal personality factor analysis that primary areas of behavioral dyscontrol, depression, abulia (apathy amotivational syndrome) anxiety reactions, and mixed psychiatric syndromes were identified among TBI survivors. Such risk factors must be kept in mind when evaluating driving potential, when formulating a risk assessment and risk management strategy, and when devising a rehabilitation or management program.

In sum, an adequate neuropsychological model would include the following criteria:

1. Delineating a hypothetical construct of "driving behavior" as a set of complex functional, dynamic behaviors. This construct would also interact dynamically with environmental and interpersonal pressures, cues, and environmental structure;

2. Would include and account for basic sensorimotor functions necessary for driving, to include medical issues which might impede, impair, or preclude "driving;"

3. Would include and account for the psychological issues related to driving risk, such as previous driving and accident/violation history, general personality and attitudinal factors, pattern and severity of alcohol/substance abuse, and the nature and extent of psychiatric disturbance;

4. Would include information processing, executive function, attentional, multi-tasking, and information processing components;

5. Would include risk identification, risk communication, and risk management/environmental strategies;

6. Would include both medical and rehabilitation as well as non-medical educational teaching, training, and management strategies.

RETURNING TO DRIVING AFTER TBI

One of the earliest "meta-analyses" of driving outcomes after TBI was provided by Hopewell and van Zomeren (1990). This included work by van Zomeren et al. (1987) that identified seven investigations that reported data on large groups of subjects with brain damage of various etiologies. These included 309 veterans of World War II who were followed 15 years after injury (Erculei, 1969) and 84 civilian subjects with between 65% and 78% of the TBI survivors being active, licensed drivers (Bijkerk et al., 1986). Two studies from rehabilitation hospitals (Koops et al., 1981; Hopewell & Price, 1985) indicated that 44–48% of TBI patients who had improved enough to be referred to a driver training program were able to resume motor vehicle operation successfully.

More recent meta-analyses have included those of Brouwer and Withaar (1997) who reviewed a number of studies and found a relicensing rate of slightly over 50% for very severe TBI patients. Failures in relicensing were found particularly to occur in patients with a very long duration of post-traumatic amnesia (exceeding 1 month), and with severe impairments of perception and judgment. The authors recommended that expanded testing should not only focus on operational capacities (eye–hand coordination and vision) but should include measures of executive functions (decision-making, multi-tasking, divided attention, judgment, impulse control, etc.) and learning potential as well.

The results of these studies, as well as the observation that the usual neuropsychological tests have only moderate success in the prediction driving skill, has led TBI researchers to the conclusion that a number of patients may be able to compensate for their residual neuropsychological impairments. Van Zomeren et al. (1987) assume that this compensation is realized by adequate decisions at the *strategic* and *tactical* levels of driving, this being a good example of *cognitive management*. For example, many TBI survivors indicated that they now drove at a lower average speed than before their injuries, would leave earlier, or would avoid inclement weather, nighttime, or freeway driving (strategic decisions). Such modifications subsequently result in a reduction of time and other pressures at the operational level, thereby reducing tactical demand.

Similarly, Schultheis et al. (2002) found that individuals with TBI who had undergone a comprehensive driver evaluation did not differ in their driving behaviors from non-TBI drivers. Specifically, the study examined both objective and subjective measures of driving behaviors occurring in the past 5 years, for 47 individuals with TBI and 22 healthy controls (HC), matched on age, gender, education, and years of driving experience. Overall, only subtle descriptive differences in driving characteristics were observed between the two groups. However, comparison of self-reported and documented reports of aberrant driving behaviors did not reveal a significantly greater number of accidents or violations among TBI participants, when compared to HC drivers. Interestingly, the findings suggested that drivers with TBI are capable of recognizing changes or difficulties in their driving capacity and were implementing compensatory strategies (Schultheis et al., 2002). That is, the results indicated that some drivers with TBI (14.9%, $n = 7$), independently elected to not return to driving after successful completion of a comprehensive driving evaluation and a substantial percentage of persons with TBI who resumed driving, reported imposing self-limitations on their driving post-injury (37.5%, $n = 15$). Similarly, when queried about unsafe driving situations, drivers with TBI reported significantly less incidents than HC, possibly suggesting less risk taking by those individuals with TBI who resumed driving.

The authors concluded that individuals with TBI, who successfully complete a comprehensive driving evaluation program, are able to re-integrate into the driving community with minimal difficulty.

DETERMINING FITNESS TO DRIVE

If up to 50% of TBI survivors are able to return to motor vehicle operations, how can such individuals be selected, what selection mechanisms may be used, and what rehabilitation strategies will aid return to driving? Faced daily with practical decision-making regarding the return of TBI survivors to driving, Hopewell and Price (1985) undertook a three-tiered study of the problem. Firstly, the investigation resulted in a rating scale based on the model used for the Brief Psychiatric Rating Scale (BPRS) (Overall & Klett, 1972, Chapter 1). Partly based upon the success of this scale as well as the author's years of experience of predicting motor vehicle operation for the US military and in civilian rehabilitation settings, the *Drivers' Neuropsychological Rating Scale*, discussed later, was ultimately developed.

Secondly, a series of 56 TBI patients who were admitted for rehabilitation and who achieved a final level of functioning equivalent to a "moderate" or "good" rating on the Glasgow Outcome Scale (Jennett & Bond, 1975) were considered for the possibility of return to motor vehicle operation, and a total of 30 (53%) of these patients were eventually able to return to motor vehicle operation. Analysis of reasons for failure to return to driving included persistent visual problems, motor difficulties necessitating assistive devices for mobility, and topographical disorientation.

Thirdly, an analysis of risk factors was performed. As pointed out by van Zomeren et al. (1987, p. 698), "Half the patients studied still ... drive. Do they present a great risk, both to themselves and to other road users?" The third portion of the investigation therefore followed the 30 patients who had returned to driving for a period of 2 years, by means of a computerized search of Texas Department of Public Safety records. Subsequently, six subjects (20%) of this group accounted for at least nine recorded accidents and seven additional moving vehicle traffic violations. Considering that 8.7% of Texas drivers between the ages of 18 and 32 (approximating the age of the experimental group) had accidents in calendar year 1985, the 20% of the TBI group having multiple subsequent accidents may constitute a high-risk population of drivers (Texas Department of Public Safety, 1985, p. 43). The existence of a high-risk cohort of TBI survivors who are potential drivers has since this original study been confirmed (Boake et al., 1998). One exception to this is the study by Schultheis et al. (2002), in which an increased risk cohort was not found upon careful follow-up. However, the participants in this latter study were all involved in an adaptive driving program, with the possibility of high-risk patients not having been referred or deselected for the program, or perhaps deselecting themselves. The other possibility exists that participation in such a program itself decreases risk.

A review of these studies suggests that the TBI driver may be viewed as a "quadruple risk," although approximately half of those improving to a "moderate" or "good" level of recovery may be expected to resume driving. First, and the most important, impaired executive functions, difficult to assess and interfering with the patient's own judgment, create the major risk factor to be addressed. Second, the preservation of over-learned motor operations, along with social/psychological pressure to resume driving, may lead to an overestimation of ability and to denial of disability by both the patient and the others. Third, this is an individual who already manifests a high level of risk based on age and gender (e.g., young male). Indeed, if the accident is due to his or her own difficulty in managing a motor vehicle, this risk has already become reality. Finally, overall reaction time has usually been slowed, also increasing correspondingly the risk factor for accident when the TBI survivor does not compensate for deficit by adopting a more cautious driving style.

The overall conclusion of these studies was that it was possible to identify which TBI patients could return to driving and that a multistage decision model was of most use in making such decisions. In addition, the importance of making some attempt to identify high-risk drivers is emphasized.

PREDICTION AND COMMUNICATION OF RISK

The assessment of driving potential of necessity dictates the concomitant evaluation of potential risk. Recent procedures have been developed which allow for relatively accurate predictions of illegal behavior, at least within reasonable time frames (Harris & Rice, 1997). These procedures are specific to different types of persons (i.e., the mentally ill, the psychopath, the sex offender). The predictive accuracy of such procedures depends on the collection of high quality objective information, both historical and current. Such models are now being used increasingly to identify and manage risk of terrorism, a goal which was not originally included in such models. In addition, risk appraisal research indicates that violence is well predictable in some populations (Monahan, 1996). Indeed, the factors most highly and consistently related to risk of violent behavior (in a general population) are historical and include age, sex, past antisocial and violent conduct, psychopathy, aggressive childhood behavior, and substance abuse. Ongoing programs of risk assessment research in psychology seek to improve the precision with which psychologists can estimate the risk of harmful behavior under specified conditions (Monahan & Steadman, 1994).

In addition to *predicting* risk, hazardous factors need to be *communicated*. Risk assessment by itself is useless if the assessment is not *communicated* and subsequently *acted upon*. An ideal system for communicating assessments of risk would provide clear, precise, and complete information regarding those assessments in a form that would be fully accessible to the parties who must make decisions and take action on the basis of those assessments. The system would also communicate this information in a manner that would reflect and facilitate the appropriate allocation and discharge of responsibilities among the participants in light of their competence and authority Schopp (1996).

And finally, the communication should ideally structure a prescriptive narrative which (1) includes a categorization of level of risk, (2) provides an estimate of time structure, and (3) communicates a prescriptive narrative. In simple terms, the communication should inform those who are responsible for completing the action plan how "bad" the risk is, when it might happen, and *what to do about it*.

CASE EXAMPLE

A middle aged Caucasian female with multifactorial brain injuries had experienced seven psychiatric hospitalizations within a period of 9 years and had been admitted to an inpatient residential brain injury rehabilitation program. Neuropsychological assessment documented her to be an extreme accident risk for the foreseeable future. She consistently stated that she wanted to drive her RV from New England to North Carolina "to be free" rather than being willing to limit her driving to therapy and necessary ADLs, and she almost injured another person when she attempted to steal a car and elope from the facility. Risk communication was provided to her family, the department of public safety (her state, Maine, mandates report and provides immunity), and her physician. A prescription was

(Continued)

CASE EXAMPLE (Continued)

provided that required the successful completion of her inpatient rehabilitation program as well as the passing of an adaptive driving program and in vivo driving test along with 1 year of successful supervised living with no psychiatric hospitalizations, drug abuse, or suicide attempts, along with compliance with the after-care program. Driving was precluded until the prescription was met, and was then limited to necessary ADLs.

POTENTIAL NEUROPSYCHOLOGICAL BATTERIES

As has been indicated, no single currently available neuropsychological "test" or "battery" is fully adequate for driving determinations, although flexible neuropsychological batteries which emphasize executive function and personality assessment seem to have the most predictive validity (Hopewell & van Zomeren, 1990). In addition, neuropsychological practice has evolved over the years from the tendency to use rigid "batteries" to the point where most clinicians favor a flexible "process" approach in which cognitive processes may be systematically evaluated. In this regard, the recent Delis-Kaplan Executive Function System (Delis et al., 2002) is designed specifically to assess executive function, and may eventually prove useful for driving determinations.

Regardless of which tests are used, rehabilitation teams should adopt a *multidimensional and multistage decision model* which also references a risk-benefit decision paradigm (Hopewell, 2002). Such a multistage decision model should be used for risk identification and management, and rehabilitation strategies then should be geared toward successfully identifying and managing those who can be rehabilitated, while at the same time identifying those who constitute a high-risk cohort, with appropriate risk management strategies and prescriptions. At the same time, some of the more psychological tests which have been used for driving determinations include the *Cognitive Behavioral Drivers Inventory,* the *Neurocognitive Driving Test,* and the *Drivers' Neuropsychological Rating Scale.*

The Cognitive Behavioral Driver's Test

This tests developed by Engum et al. (1988a) includes several visual attention tasks and is designed to work in conjunction with standardized neuropsychological measures, including the Trail Making Tests and subtests of the WAIS. Engum et al. (1990) administered *The Cognitive Behavioral Drivers Inventory* to 232 rehabilitation patients with cerebral vascular accidents, traumatic head injuries, spinal cord injuries, and other neurological disorders (e.g., multiple sclerosis, Alzheimer's disease, Parkinson's disease) to restandardize the normative tables and enhance the rigor and precision of the decision-making process. This test has often been used as an aid to help with driving decisions, but is limited due to the emphasis upon general cognitive as opposed to executive and personality functions. A General Driver's Index is provided, and the work of Engum et al., has helped to establish normative tables and guidelines for rehabilitative professionals seeking to evaluate the operational driving skills of their brain-injured patients.

The Neurocognitive Driving Test

Developed by Schultheis (1998), the Neurocognitive Driving Test was designed to address four critical factors needed for accurate evaluation of cognitively impaired individuals: (1) the need for ecologically valid tests, (2) the need for objective measures of cognitive skills related to driving, (3) the need for practical, user-friendly tools, and (4) the need to incorporate theoretical rationale to the development of assessment tools. Based on Michon's Hierarchical Model of Driving Tasks and through the use of the Power Laboratory (Chute & Westall, 1996), this computerized program allows assessment of driving-related behaviors in ecologically valid tasks and situations. The program is divided into four computerized tasks: (1) assessment of pre-driving behaviors, (2) reaction time, (3) visual fields, and (4) performance in four real-life driving scenarios.

The first component of the *Neurocognitive Driving Test*, the Pre-Driving Task, targets an individual's ability to identify correctly the important information needed prior to engaging in driving. This includes task such as, route planning, time management, awareness of automotive needs, and identification of one's ability to drive. The Reaction Time Task provides measures of simple and choice reaction time by measuring the subject's response time to an identified stimulus. The Visual Field Task provides measures of the subject's left and right visual fields. The Driving Scenario Task consists of four "real-life" complex driving situations. The "virtual reality-like" driving scenarios movies include following signs, following verbal directions, following written directions, and an emergency situation (fire engine in your path).

Current advances in technology have allowed these researchers to update this program to a virtual reality-based driving simulation program (Schultheis and Mourant, 2001). Studies to date have demonstrated that VR can provide objective and novel measurements of complex behaviors, such as driving. Preliminary findings from studies examining concurrent validity of performance of individuals with and without brain injury indicate that the VRDS driving performance measures are related to cognitive domains identified as relevant to driving (Schultheis et al., 2004; Schultheis et al., 2006).

The Drivers' Neuropsychological Rating Scale

Developed in 1997 by Hopewell, the Driver's Neuropsychological Rating Scale was designed to fulfill a need for the rating of risk assessment as well as the planning of rehabilitation strategies by rehabilitation teams working within a mental health, rehabilitation, or geriatric framework. It was not designed to be a standardized psychometric instrument, but rather was intended to be a rating guide used by rehabilitation and mental health professionals with an understanding of psychiatric as well as medical and neurological disorders. As a rating guide, the scale was not designed to be used in a rigid manner, but should be used by rehabilitation teams as an ongoing aid to risk assessment, risk communication, decision-making, and the development of rehabilitation and safety strategies. The test can therefore be used as a component of multidisciplinary assessment and can make use of practically any available testing measure, although it may also be used by individual clinicians. This consists of 15 separate categories requiring specific rating by the clinician filling out the protocol, to include (1) Visual Status; (2) Hearing Screening; (3) Active Range of Motion; (4) Functional Strength; (5) Reaction Time Assessment; (6) Cognitive Status; (7) Executive Functioning; (8) Aggressive Behaviors; (9) Criminal and Driving History; (10) Psychiatric History; (11) Substance Abuse History; (12) Independent Living Skills; (13) Safety Awareness Skills; (14) Compliance Issues, and (15) Health Risks.

The model of risk assessment includes four categorical levels: Category I: Low Crash Risk; Category II: Moderate Crash Risk; Category III: High Crash Risk; and Category IV: Extreme Crash Risk. Communication of the risk category provides both a narrative description as well as a narrative recommended prescriptive action, both of which lay the foundation for further rehabilitation and a strategy for returning to driving.

Two hundred and thirty-seven (237) brain-injured clients were rated on both the brain injury modification of the *Katz Adjustment Scale* (Jackson et al., 1992) and the *Driver's Neuropsychological Rating Scale* (Hopewell, 1997). Inter-tester reliability for the Ph.D. level raters ranged from 0.71 to 0.84, while the inter-tester reliability for the Master's and Bachelor's level psychology graduates ranged from 0.57 to 0.78. A Chi-Square analysis $=67.10$, which demonstrated a high degree of predictive validity between those brain-injured clients who had been allowed to return to motor vehicle operations or who had perhaps never stopped (driving cohort) and those whose driving privileges had been rescinded at the time of the examination (not driving).

DRIVER REHABILITATION STRATEGIES

Cognitive retraining or rehabilitation is primarily based upon a skill acquisition model, with the goal of aiding the recovery process by improving cognitive function, regaining or retraining cognitive skills, and increasing overall levels of cognitive functioning and stamina. Such "retraining" generally consists of efforts to improve certain specific aspects of complex cognitive processes, such as focused attention or speed of information processing, and, when possible, of finding methods to help the patient compensate for or supplement lost abilities. Although the term "cognitive rehabilitation" is often used, this retraining model also includes strategies to improve psychological and behavioral functioning, such as increased prosocial skills, increased behavioral stamina and stability, increased motivation and initiation, improved insight and self-monitoring, and decreased aggression and inappropriate behavior.

Cognitive management, on the other hand, does not purport to restore lost higher cerebral functions, but is designed to help the patient as well as family members, authorities such as employers and regulatory officials and therapists to understand the severity and nature of impaired cognitive processes, as well as the anticipated recovery process. In addition, *cognitive management* provides management of the environment as well as management of task demands such as speed of return to work and a graduated transition for work or school return, appropriate management of cognitive demands, and consultation with family, employer, or school authorities regarding the appropriate management of such environmental demands.

Efforts for improving cognitive function using cognitive rehabilitation strategies have primarily focused on functions of alertness, attentional processes, visual scanning and visual perception, language function, memory skills, executive function, and topographical orientation. However, one fruitful area of remediation is that of visual scanning and visual capacity during driving tasks. Occupational therapists are increasingly called upon to work with visually impaired clients in rehabilitation attempts. However, Klavora et al. (1995) have felt that a number of conventional rehabilitation exercises, such as pencil-and-paper and computer tasks, do not train perceptual and motor skills as applied to a complex, multi-skill activity such as driving. The investigators examined the usefulness of the Dynavision apparatus for driving-related rehabilitation, and results suggested that that such training resulted in significantly improved behind-the-wheel driving assessments. Comparisons between pretests, posttests, and follow-up tests on a number of Dynavision, response, and reaction time variables showed significant improvements and maintenance effects. Dynavision performance, and, to a lesser extent, choice visual reaction and response times, were found to differentiate between persons assessed as safe and unsafe to drive, and between older and younger drivers.

Increasingly, the *Useful Field of View Test* (UFOV) is being used as a measure of the functional or useful range of peripheral vision under cognitive load conditions (Fisk et al., 2002). As cognitive load is increased by increasing task complexity, the functional range of peripheral vision (i.e., the degree of peripheral vision from which information is processed) becomes restricted. The UFOV is increasingly used to assess as well as help in planning remediation programs for visual disorders seen with TBI which impeded driving.

In contrast to the "cognitive functions," it is the personality, behavioral, and emotional changes which have been recognized as frequently being the most handicapping sequelae of TBI by many psychological investigators. Such problems create the greatest burden for the family and long-term caregivers (Lezak, 1978; Oddy et al., 1978) and are the major preventative factor in return to employment or driving status.

In considering cognitive management strategies, driving behavior in traffic may be regarded as a hierarchically organized set of tasks with three levels: strategic, tactical, and operational (Michon, 1979). At the strategic level, driving decisions are generally made without time pressure and involve choices such as route to be taken and time of day driving will occur. Tactical decisions are made on the road, involve slight time pressure, and usually involve judgments such as when to slow down or switch on headlights during periods of poor visibility. This level of functioning especially requires the ability to foresee, anticipate, and judge consequences. The operational level involves numerous perceptions and actions during driving and contains a constant demand of time pressure. Salient identified operational problems include poor visual scanning, spatial and orientation dysfunction, poor tracking, motor retardation, confusion in complex or simultaneous demand situations, and poor coordination of the lower extremities (van Zomeren et al., 1987).

An important aspect of this three-level model is contained in a concept of a hierarchical structure, thus providing the basis for cognitive management strategies. To a large extent, decisions on a higher level determine the workload on lower levels. For example, the strategic decision to avoid rush-hour traffic will result in fewer decisions and actions to be taken at the tactical and operational levels. Likewise, the tactical decision to increase speed will place higher demands on the operational level in terms of tracking ability, quick responses to unexpected situations, and the like. This hierarchical nature can also be referred to as *top-down control*. In general, cognitive management strategies also comprise components such as: Pacing (adjusting the speed of task demands, number of tasks or reduction of multi-tasking, or adjustment of information input in order to achieve success); Selection of tasks and number of tasks; Selection of task complexity or level of difficulty; Use of time out and stress management procedures; and use of cueing and/or assistive devices.

Environmental management overlaps somewhat with executive/cognitive function management and may be divided into *environmental structure* and *target hardening* strategies. Environmental structure includes items meant to provide either a more user-friendly or user-safe environment and could include strategies such as improving mirror capability or ergonomic functions such as clearly read and unambiguous panel symbols.

Target hardening includes environmental structure or modifications which increase safety or decrease driving risk by direct manipulation of the potential accident target. Examples would include the purchase of a car with increase crash resistant features such as airbags, side-impact panels, global positioning capability, easy-to-use seatbelts, installation of fuel tank firewalls or "fuel cells" to prevent gasoline spraying into the back seat in the event of a rear end collision, etc. As an example of such target hardening, a TBI survivor might well select a vehicle with a high-safety rating as opposed to choosing to return to driving by operating a motorcycle without a helmet, a seemingly common-sense decision, but one which may be encountered more frequently than would be expected with this population.

Finally, the increase in rehabilitation cases such as the expansion of brain injury programs as well as other medical advances as reviewed above has led to a steady extension of adaptive driving programs around the country. Jones et al. (1983) for example, described an early hospital driving assessment and training program implemented in 1977 for outpatients experiencing residual impairment from brain damage. Assessment by an occupational therapist consisted of an on-road test and several off-road tests (i.e., vision, reaction, computerized preview tracking, general physical/psychological appraisal) but did not include a neuropsychological component, thereby being an example of a driving skill model.

Fox et al. (1992) illustrated the Coorabel Driver Assessment and Training Program which incorporated assessments by a medical practitioner, a neuropsychologist, an occupational therapist and a driving instructor, along with both off- and on-road examinations. One hundred and twenty-nine (129) consecutive referrals were reviewed. In 47 cases the medical practitioner was unable to make a final decision regarding driver competence, substantiating the consensus of investigators that motor vehicle operation is not a medical condition but a functional behavior which is best addressed by psychological methods. Neuropsychological and on-road assessments resulted in definitive decisions for 39 of these 47 cases. It was suggested that multidisciplinary assessment of driver competence, inclusive of on-road testing, is essential, as medical guidelines alone are insufficient to predict driver fitness.

SIMULATOR TRAINING

A number of computer programs as well as small vehicular simulators have been used to investigate driving skill and rehabilitation. There has been some evidence to show that training in small vehicle simulators may produce a therapeutic effect (Sivak et al., 1984; Kewman et al., 1985; Hale et al., 1987; Gianutsos, 1994; Galski et al., 1997). However, the question of how much simulators have in common with standard size vehicles as well as how computer training generalizes to in vivo tasks continues to be posed. Many investigators have concluded that computer simulators currently have only moderate predictive ability for actual motor vehicle operation, and they appear to be most useful in training specific skills or in helping patients, families, or staff gain insight into neuropsychological deficits which would preclude driving. For example, Timm and Hokendorf (1994) found that an individual's driving fitness could not be diagnosed on the basis of laboratory testing alone. They felt that the deficits elicited by the tests had to be verified concerning their impact in real road traffic in every individual case. In our brain injury laboratories, we have often found it helpful to allow patients who are unquestionably unable to drive, and yet who demonstrate strong, most likely organically based denial, to work with the simulator to help with insight. However, since the ultimate goal is to return the driver to functional vehicle operation, on-road assessment and training remain the final criteria for adaptive driving programs, and should be used in conjunction with simulator programs, not in lieu of them, if such program are available. Most adaptive driving programs still make use of in vivo on-the-road assessment and training in addition to simulator use. Some of the limitations of in vivo programs, however, include a possible lack of test complexity, possible increased risk to driver and public, and cost (Galski et al., 2000).

PHARMACOLOGICAL MANAGEMENT

Psychopharmacological management with potential TBI drivers falls into two related categories. First, as many patients may be treated with some type of psychotropic medication, adverse drug reactions (ADRs) associated with such treatment which may interfere with or preclude driving must be identified, monitored, and avoided or at least minimized if possible. Secondly, the newer medications in particular are known to aid more specifically in returning brain neurotransmitter levels and function to more normal levels, and therapeutic medications which may improve and/or normalize brain function may be very desirable.

As Lemoine and Ohayon (1996) remind us, the responsibility of psychotropic drugs as a cause of road traffic accidents remains difficult to evaluate with precision, and the accident rate associated with ADRs among TBI survivors is essentially unknown. Different studies performed in a variety of countries provide a certain precision in relation to percentage of injured drivers whose blood contained psychotropic substances (8–10% according to studies reviewed by the authors). On the other hand, the authors assert that it is practically impossible to really know whether these products were or were not the cause of the accidents because underlying or associated pathologies can equally create problems such as lack of attention and other vigilance deficits. There also remains the possibility of suicidal or aggressive tendencies, also not unknown among TBI survivors. Available medications able to create or exacerbate such problems are numerous and their mechanisms of action vary considerably, being able to influence vision, impulsiveness, and vigilance. Such medications can act either by direct mechanisms of sedation or through secondary metabolic mechanisms.

For the most part, the worrisome medications belong to the different classes of sedative medicines: the benzodiazepines, antiepileptics, some antihistaminic agents, some antidepressants, some thymo-regulators, and some anti-hypertensives. Also included are disinhibitors or stimulant classes such as amphetamines and related drugs, caffeine and codeine. Some medications, such as codeine and anticholinergic drugs can also easily be abused. In addition, "natural" and herbal agents are becoming so increasingly popular that their possible us should never be excluded, and many of these agents may present with substantial anticholinergic, sedative depressant, or agitating effects, all of which could be catastrophic for a TBI survivor (De La Cancela & Hopewell, 1999). Lemoine and Ohayon (1996) feel that it may be methodologically impossible for research ever precisely to quantify the share of responsibility carried by psychotropic drugs in causing road traffic accidents, but they feel that this relationship remains "highly probable." In addition, many TBI survivors may be prone to alcohol or other substance abuse as co-morbid disorders, at times trying to self-medicate, and such substance abuse would well be expected to interact with many prescribed psychotropics. The same appears to be increasingly true for the use of "natural" or herbal substances, some of which may have very potent effects and substantial interactions (De La Cancela & Hopewell, 1999). Health care professionals who provide medication management for TBI survivors, these now including prescribing psychologists, and who may treat many such patients who are driving, should therefore regularly stay advised of such risks and provide adequate and ongoing monitoring of all prescription and substance use in this population.

THE THERAPEUTIC ASPECTS OF
PSYCHOTROPICS

When considering treatment of brain injury, especially the use of pharmacological agents, it must also be remembered that brain injury invariably radically alters the function of the brain, and not just its *structure*. Brain injury studies frequently review the structural damage caused by acceleration/deceleration injuries, penetrating brain injuries, and other such injuries. Often mentioned are the neurobehavioral effects of selective injuries to the frontal and temporal poles, axonal shearing, damage to the memory and affective brain centers, and damage due to differential tissue density, etc., with many neurobehavioral disturbances resulting from loss of neural tissue. However, it is important to remember that the brain cannot work properly without concomitantly being able to maintain the *functional* integrity of the underlying neurotransmitter systems. Recent evidence that pharmacological treatment such as treatment with antidepressants results in long-term structural brain changes also suggests that pharmacotherapy should not be considered simply as a *management* strategy, but may well be a genuine *rehabilitation* strategy (Drevets, 1998).

Typical Psychopharmacological Agents Used in TBI

The psychopharmacological agents currently found to be useful in treating brain injury generally fall into the following classes, although other agents may also be of some use: (1) antidepressants, (2) neuroleptics/antipsychotics, (3) mood stabilizers/neuromodulators, (4) alpha/beta blockers, (5) stimulants, (6) benzodiazepines, and (7) cognitive enhancers and neuroprotective agents. Hallucinogenics and the sedative/hypnotics are of little use or are contraindicated with the TBI population, and are generally avoided when possible. Also, as has been noted, the increasingly prevalent use of "natural" and herbal agents is of considerable importance and cannot be ignored by physicians or prescribing psychologists (for a more comprehensive discussion of pharmacological agents see chapter 10).

In summary, medication management for the TBI survivor is often found to be necessary, and targets symptom management on a long-term basis rather than being "restorative" or "curative." Although useful and at times critical, pharmacological management is not to be used solely in lieu of behavioral intervention and counseling, but *concomitantly* with such interventions. In addition, pharmacological management is not to be viewed as some type of "cognitive cure," neither is it to be used for purposes of chemical restraint except in emergency situations.

As Stahl (1996) has pointed out, perhaps psychopharmacological treatments for cognitive disorders in the future will need to borrow a chapter out of the book of cancer chemotherapy. In cancer chemotherapy, the standard of treatment is to use multiple drugs simultaneously. "Combination chemotherapy" for malignancy utilizes the approach of adding together several independent therapeutic mechanisms. As noted, the newer pharmacological agents may be potentially more helpful for TBI survivors because they are better tolerated, have better side effect profiles, and some demonstrate better efficacy. However, TBI survivors may well have limited access to these agents, especially as managed profit companies which ration care or state agencies may not allow the newer and more expensive agents to be prescribed as financial costs are placed above human costs. Education of providers and patients, policy changes in the public sector, wider implementation of research policies concerning TBI survivors, and different marketing strategies by pharmaceutical concerns are probably necessary to maximize pharmacotherapy benefit to patient groups. Side effects which may interfere with driving, and the use of "natural" or herbal agents should be monitored closely and discontinued or modified if problematic.

CONCLUSIONS

A number of overall conclusions from 40 years of driving and rehabilitation studies can now be summarized with relative certainty. Approximately half of TBI survivors may eventually return to motor vehicle operations, with appropriate rehabilitation and driving restrictions/modifications. A cohort of such rehabilitated drivers, however, may manifest a higher risk level than non-clinical drivers even if they are able to return to driving, and this group of drivers may need additional monitoring or intervention. Successful return to driving seems to depend on good awareness and early identification of driving problems, competent medical/psychiatric management and rehabilitation, effective domain-specific education, and adequate motivation and compliance. Simple predictive tests, a medical model by itself, or simply a driving skill model of prediction are insufficient in the assessment of driving capability. Rather, a neuropsychological model which incorporates a review of driving history, the assessment of complex neuropsychological and executive functioning, and in vivo testing along with currently accepted concepts of risk identification and risk management are necessary along with adequate medical management and adaptive driving rehabilitation is preferred. Multistage decision models should be used for risk identification and management, and currently accepted risk identification and management strategies can be successfully employed. Such strategies should be geared toward successfully identifying and managing those who can be rehabilitated, and identifying those who constitute a high-risk cohort. Medication management may be an integral part of the overall rehabilitation process, and many new pharmacological agents show increasing promise in terms of aiding cognitive and affective function. However, medications should be monitored carefully to avoid ADRs or interactions which may increase risk, along with the concomitant use of "natural" or herbal agents which may be problematic. Alcohol and illicit substance use should of course, be eschewed.

REFERENCES

Bijkerk, M., Brouwer, W. H., & van Zomeren, A. H. (1986). *Contusio cerebri-jarenlange kopzorgen?* Groningen, Netherlands: State University, Internal Report Department of Clinical Psychology.

Boake, C., MacLeod, M., High, Jr. W. M., & Lehmkuhl, L. D. (1998b, February). Increased risk of motor vehicle crashes among drivers with traumatic brain injury. Paper presented at the 26th Annual Meeting of the International Neuropsychological Society, Honolulu, HI. *J. Int. Neuropsychol. Soc.*, 4, 75.

Brouwer, W. H., & Withaar, F. K. (1997 Jul). Fitness to drive after traumatic brain injury. *Neuropsychol. Rehabil.*, 7(3), 177–193.

Brouwer, W. H., Witbaar, F. K., Tant, M. L. M., & van Zomeren, A. H. (2002 Feb). Attention and driving in traumatic brain injury: A question of coping with time-pressure. *J. Head Trauma Rehabil.*, 17(1), 1–15.

Center for Disease Control. (2006). Atlanta.

Chute, D., & Westall, R. (1996). *B/C Power Laboratory*. New York: Brooks/Cole Publishing Company.

Coleman, R. D., Rapport, L. J., Ergh, T. C., Hanks, R. A., Ricker, J. H., & Millis, S. R. (2002). Predictors of driving outcome after traumatic brain injury. *Arch Phys Med Rehabil.*, 83, 1415–1422.

Cremona, A. (1986). Mad drivers: Psychiatric illness and driving performance. *Br. J. Hosp. Medirille*, 193–195.

Dawson, D. R., & Chipman, M. (1995). The Disablement Experienced by Traumatically Brain-Injured Adults Living in the Community. *Brain Inj.*, 9(4), 339–353.

De La Cancela, V., & Hopewell, C. A. (1999). Ethnocultural competence in the prescribing of psychotropic medications. *Am. J. Psychopharmacol.*, 2, 454–455.

Devani Serio, C., & Devens, M. (1994). Employment problems following traumatic brain injury: families assess the cause. *Neurorehabilitation*, 4, 53–57.

Delis, D. C., Kaplan, E., & Kramer, J. H. (2002). *Delis-Kaplan Executive Functional System*. San Antonio, Texas: The Psychological Corporation.

Drevets, Wayne C., & Raichle, Marcus E. (1998). Reciprocal suppression of regional cerebral blood flow during emotional versus higher cognitive processes: Implications for interactions between emotion and cognition. *Cognition & Emotion*, 12(3), 353–385.

Engum, E. S., & Lambert, E. W. (1990). Restandardization of the cognitive behavioral driver's inventory. *Cognitive Rehabilitation*, 8, 20–27.

Engum, E. S., Pendergrass, T. M., Cron, L., Lambert, E. W., & Hulse, C. K. (1988a). Cognitive behavioral driver's inventory. *Cognitive Rehabilitation*, 6, 34–48.

Engum, E. S., Lambert, E. W., Womac, J., & Pendergrass, T. (1988b). Norms and decision making rules for the Cognitive Behavioral Driver's Inventory. *Cognitive Rehabilitation* (November/December), 12–18.

Erculei, F. (1969). The socio-economic rehabilitation of head-injured men. In: A. E. Walker, W. F. Caveness, & M. Critchley (Eds.), *The Late Effects of Head Injury*. Springfield, IL: Charles C. Thomas.

Fisk, G. D., Schneider, J. J., & Novack, T. A. (1998 Aug). Driving following traumatic brain injury: Prevalence, exposure, advice and evaluations. *Brain Injury*, 12(8), 683–695.

Fisk, G. D., Novack, T., Mennemeier, M., & Roenker, D. (2002 Feb). Useful field of view after traumatic brain injury. *J. Head Trauma Rehabil.*, 17(1), 16–25.

Formisano, R., Bivona, U., Brunelli, S., Giustini, M., Longo, E., & Taggi, F. (2005). A preliminary investigation of road traffic accident rate after severe brain injury. *Brain Inj.*, 19(3), 159–163.

Fox, G. K., Bashford, G. M., & Caust, S. L. (1992). Identifying safe versus unsafe drivers following brain impairment: The Coorabel Programme. *Disabil. Rehabil.*, 14(3), 140–145.

Galski, T., Bruno, R. L., & Ehle, H. T. (1993). Prediction of behind-the-wheel driving performance in patients with cerebral brain damage: a discriminant function analysis. *Am J Occup Ther.*, 47(5), 391–396.

Galski, T., Ehle, H. T., & Williams, J. B. (1997). Off-road driving evaluations for persons with cerebral injury: A factor analytic study of predriver and simulator testing. *Am. J. Occup. Ther.*, *51*(5), 352–359.

Galski, T., Ehle, H. T., McDonald, M. A., & Mackevic, J. (2000). Evaluating Fitness to Drive after Cerebral Injury: Basic Issues and Recommendations for Medical and Legal Communities. *Journal of Head Trauma Rehabilitation*, *15*(3), 895–908.

Garretson, M., & Peck, R. C. (1982). Factors associated with fatal accident involvement among California drivers. *J. Saf. Res.*, *13*, 141–156.

Gianutsos, R. (1994). Driving advisement with the Elemental Driving Simulator (EDS): When less suffices. *Behav. Res. Meth. Instrum. Comput.*, *26*(2), 183–186.

Gouvier, W. D., Maxfield, M. W., Schwietzer, J. R., Horton, C. R., Slipp, M., Neilson, K., & Hale, P. N. (1989). Psychometric prediction of driving performance among the disabled. *Arch. Phys. Med. Rehabil.*, *70*, 745–750.

Greenshields, B. D., & Platt, F. N. (1967). Development of a method of predicting high-accident and high-violation drivers. *J. Appl. Psychol.*, *51*(3), 205–210.

Hale, Jr. P. N. (1986–1987). Rehabilitation engineering for personal licensed vehicles (Annual Report). Ruston, Louisiana: *The Center for Rehabilitation Science and Biomedical Engineering.*

Hale, P. N., Schweitzer, J. R., Shipp, M., & Gouvier, W. D. (1987). A small-scale vehicle for assessing and training driving skills among the disabled. *Arch. Phys. Med. Rehabil.*, *68*, 741–742.

Harano, R. M., Peck, R. C., & McBride, R. S. (1975). The prediction of accident liability through biographical data and psychometric tests. *J. Saf. Res.*, *7*(1), 16–52.

Harris, G. T., & Rice, M. E. (1997). An overview of research on the prediction of dangerousness. *Psychiatr. Serv.*, *48*(9 Sep), 1168–1176.

Hawley, C. A. (2001). Returning to driving after head injury. *Journal of Neurology, Neurosurgery, and Psychiatry*, *70*, 761–766.

Heaton, R. K., & Pendleton, M. G. (1981). Use of neuropsychological tests to predict adult patients' everyday functioning. *J. Consult. Clin. Psychol.*, *49*, 807–821.

Hopewell, C. A. (1997). The drivers' neuropsychological rating scale. San Diego: International Mental Health Network. ISBN 1-58028-057-9

Hopewell, C. A. (2002). Driving assessment issues for practicing clinicians. *J. Head Trauma Rehabil.*, *17*(1), 48–61.

Hopewell, C. A., & Price, R. J. (1985). Driving after head injury. *J. Clin. Exp. Neuropsychol.*, *7*, 148.

Hopewell, C. A., & van Zomeren, A. H. (1990). Neuropsychological aspects of motor vehicle operation. In: D. E. Tupper, & K. D. Cicerone (Eds.), *The Neuropsychology of Everyday Life: Assessment and Basic Competencies.* Boston: Kluwer.

Jackson, H. F., Hopewell, C. A., Glass, C. A., Warburg, R., Dewey, M., & Ghadliali, E. (1992). The Katz Adjustment Scale: Modification for use with survivors of traumatic brain injury and spinal injury. *Brain Injury*, *6*(2), 109–127.

Jennett, B., & Bond, M. (1975). Assessment of outcome after severe brain damage. *Lancet*, *1*, 480–487.

Jones, R., Giddens, H., & Croft, D. (1983). Assessment and training of brain-damaged drivers. *Am J Occup Ther.*, *37*(11), 754–760.

Kewman, D. G., Seigerman, C., Kintner, H., & Reeder, C. (1985). Simulation training of psychomotor skills: Teaching the brain injured to drive. *Rehabil. Psychol.*, *30*(1), 11–27.

Klavora, P., Gaskovski, P., Martin, K., Forsyth, R. D., Heslegrave, R. J., Young, M., & Quinn, R. P. (1995). The effects of Dynavision rehabilitation on behind-the-wheel driving ability and selected psychomotor abilities of persons after stroke. *Am. J. Occup. Ther.*, *49*(6), 534–542.

Koops, D., Deelman, B. G., & Saan, R. J. (1981). *He leven na een onusio erebri – een onderzoek onder 50 traumapatienten.* Groningen, Netherlands: State University, Internal Report Department of Neuropsychology.

Lemoine, P., & Ohayon, M. (1996). Abuse of psychotropic drugs during driving. *Encephale*, *22*(1), 1–6.

Lengenfelder, J., Schultheis, M. T., Al-Shihabi, T., Mourant, R., & DeLuca, J. (2002). Divided attention and driving: A pilot study using virtual reality technology. *J. Head Trauma Rehabil.*, *17*, 26–37.

Lezak, M. D. (1978). Living with the characterologically altered brain injured patient. *J Clin Psychiatry*, *39*(7), 592–598.

Marottoli, R. A., Mendes de Leon, C. F., Glass, T. A., Williams, C. S., Cooney, L. M. Jr, Berkman, L. F., & Tinetti, M. E. (1997). Driving cessation and increased depressive symptoms: prospective evidence from the New Haven EPESE. Established Populations for Epidemiologic Studies of the Elderly. *J Am Geriatr Soc.*, *45*(2), 202–206.

McFarland, R. A., Moore, R. C., & Warren, A. B. (1954). *Human Variables in Motor Vehicle Accidents: A Review of the Literature*. Cambridge, MA: Harvard School of Public Health.

Michon, J. A. (1979). Dealing with danger. Unpublished manuscript. Groningen, Netherlands: State University, Traffic Research Center.

Michon, J. A. (1985). A critical view of driver behavior models: What do we know, what should we do? In: L. Evans, & R. C. Schwing (Eds.), *Human Behavior and Traffic Safety* (pp. 485–520). New York: Plenum Press.

Mihal, W. L., & Barrett, G. V. (1976). Individual differences in perceptual information processing and their relation to automobile accident involvement. *J. Appl. Psychol.*, *61*(2), 229–233.

Miller, T. M., & Schuster, D. H. (1983). Long-term predictability of driver behavior. *Accid. Anal. Prev.*, *15*(1), 11–22.

Monahan, J. (1996 Mar). Risk appraisal and management of violent behavior. *Crim. Justice Behav.*, *23*(1), 107–120.

Monahan, J., & Steadman, H. (1994). *Violence and Mental Disorder: Developments in Risk Assessment*. Chicago: University of Chicago Press.

Noyes, R. Jr. (1985). Motor vehicle accidents related to psychiatric impairment. *Psychosomatics*, *26*(7), 569–580.

Oddy, M., Humphrey, M., & Uttley, D. (1978). Stresses upon the relatives of head injury patients. *Br. J. Psychiatr.*, *133*, 507–513.

Overall, J. E., & Klett, C. J. (1972). *Applied Multivariate Analysis*. New York: McGraw-Hill.

Parasuraman, R., & Nestor, P. (1993). Attention and driving. Assessment in elderly individuals with dementia. Clin Geriatr Med., *9*(2), 377–387.

Peck, R. C., & Kuan, J. (1983). A statistical model of individual accident risk prediction using driver record territory and other biographical factors. *Accid. Anal. Prev.*, *15*(5), 371–393.

Pettis, R. W. (1992). Tarasoff and the dangerous driver: a look at the driving cases. *Bull Am Acad Psychiatry Law*, *20*(4), 427–437.

Pietrapiana, P., Tamietto, M., Torrini, G., Mezzanato, T., Rago, R., & Perino, C. (2005). Role of premorbid factors in predicting safe return to driving after severe TBI. *Brain Inj.*, *19*(3), 197–211.

Rapport, L., Hanks, R., & Bryer, R. (2006). Barriers to Driving and Community Integration After Traumatic Brain Injury. *Journal of Head Trauma Rehabilitation*, *21*(1), 34–44.

Rao, V., & Lyketsos, C. G. (2002). Psychiatric aspects of traumatic brain injury. (J. L. Levenson, C. G. Lyketsos, & P. T. Trzepacz, Eds.) Psychiatry In The Medically Ill; *The Psychiatric Clinics Of North America*, Volume 25, Number I, March, 43–69.

Schuster, D. H. (1968). Prediction of follow-up driving accidents and violations. *Res. Rev.* (March), 17–21.

Schultheis, M. T. (1998 Dec). PhD Thesis, Drexel University, Philadelphia, PA.

Schultheis, M. T., & Mourant, R. R. (2001). Virtual Reality and Driving: The Road to Better Assessment of Cognitively Impaired Populations. *Presence: Teleoperators and Virtual Environments*, *10*(4), 436–444.

Schultheis, M., Matheis, R. J., Nead, R., & DeLuca, J. (2002 Feb). Driving behaviors following brain injury: Self-report and motor vehicle records. *J. Head Trauma Rehabil.*, *17*(1), 38–47.

Schultheis, M. T., Rebimbas, J., Ni, A., Edwards, W. T., DeLuca, J., & Millis, S. R. (2004). Driving and acquired brain injury: The cognitive correlates of speed management in a virtual environment. *Archives of Clinical Neuropsychology*, *19*(7), 905.

Schultheis, M. T., Simone, L. K., Roseman, E., Nead, R., Rebimbas, J., & Mourant, R. (2006). Stopping behavior in a VR driving simulator: A new clinical measure for the assessment of driving? *IEEE-Engineering in Medicine & Biological Science*, 4921–4924.

Selzer, M. L., Rogers, J. E., & Kern, S. (1968 Feb). Fatal accidents: The role of psychopathology, social stress, and acute disturbance. *Am. J. Psychiatr.*, *124*(8), 46–54.

Sivak, M., Hill, C. S., & Olson, P. L. (1984). Computerized video tasks as training techniques for driving-related perceptual deficits of persons with brain damage: A pilot evaluation. *Int. J. Rehabil. Res.*, *7*(4), 389–398.

Stahl, S. (1996). Mechanism of action of serotonin selective reuptake inhibitors serotonin receptors and pathways mediate therapeutic effects and side effects. *J. Affective Disorders*, *51*(3), 215–235.

Stokx, L. C., & Gaillard, A. W. (1986). Task and driving performance of patients with a severe concussion of the brain. *Journal of Clinical and Experimental Neuropsychology*, *8*(4), 421–436.

Texas Department of Public Safety (1985). *Motor Vehicle Traffic Accidents*. Austin: Texas Department of Public Safety.

Timm, H., & Hokendorf, H. (1994). Possibilities of driver fitness diagnosis and training using a stationary training car. *Rehabilitation (Stuttg)*, *33*(4), 237–241.

Tsuang, M. T., Boor, M., & Fleming, J. A. (1985). Psychiatric aspects of traffic accidents. *Am. J. Psychiatr.*, *142*(5), 538–546.

Wallace, J. E., & Crancer, A. (1971). Licensing exams and their relation to subsequent driving record. *Behav. Res. Highway Saf.*, *2*, 53–65.

6

DRIVING AND THE

DEMENTIAS

GILLIAN K. FOX, ALAN HOPEWELL,
EMILY ROSEMAN AND MARIA T. SCHULTHEIS

INTRODUCTION

The number of older drivers and their mileage each year has increased (Ball et al., 1998). The number of older drivers with dementia is also increasing. Without doubt, the dementing conditions are among the most problematic faced by our aging drivers. In addition to affecting cognitive and visuomotor abilities that can impact everyday activities, such as driving; the dementing illnesses can also deprive individuals of the very judgment and insight needed to assess accurately declining abilities and increasing risk due to these deficits. At the same time, many dementing conditions are progressive and tend to be insidious, making detection more difficult for patients, families, and health care professionals.

Alzheimer's disease (AD), the most common cause of dementia, has been estimated to affect as many as 11.6% of those aged 65 and older, and 47.8% of those aged 85 and older (Evans et al., 1989). AD is steadily progressive and characterized by a variety of cognitive function abnormalities, which may have a negative impact on everyday activities including driving. Competence in driving a motor vehicle has implications both for the safety of the individual affected by dementia and for other road users. Accordingly, questions frequently encountered by health care providers include whether individuals with dementia are able to continue to drive, and when they should stop driving. Because of the high prevalence of AD over other dementias, the current chapter will focus predominantly on AD and driving. However, it is important to note, that much of the past research examining dementia and driving includes mixed samples, which have served to identify common driving difficulties among this population. Additionally, much work examining driving among healthy older drivers overlaps with this domain. This chapter will include an overview of driving and dementia, followed by a review of current driving assessment approaches. A brief review of other dementias and driving will also be presented.

OVERVIEW

The actual public health risk of drivers with dementia is unknown. While it has been observed that drivers with dementia generally drive fewer miles and frequently voluntarily cease driving, there is also evidence that some drivers with dementia have insufficient self monitoring to reliably stop driving when they are demonstrating at risk driving behaviors (Morris, 1997). Tests of visual acuity and peripheral vision, as used in driver licensing, are not adequate to identify which individual older drivers are more likely to be involved in crashes (Ball, 1997), although state-mandated tests of visual acuity at license renewal have been found to be associated with lower fatal crash risk for elderly drivers (Levy et al., 1995).

Retrospective surveys concerning driving suggest that many patients diagnosed with dementia do continue to drive and may be reluctant to give up driving, and also have a higher risk of crashes (Friedland et al., 1988; Lucas-Blaustein et al., 1988; Gilley et al., 1991; Dubinsky et al., 1992; Logsdon et al., 1992; Tuokko et al., 1995). It is noteworthy that two retrospective studies found that only 50% of drivers with AD had ceased driving within a 3-year period from onset of dementia (Friedland et al., 1988; Drachman & Swearer, 1993), after which time crash risk increases substantially. Two retrospective studies (Friedland et al., 1988; Lucas-Blaustein et al., 1988) recommended that a diagnosis of AD preclude continuation of driving. However, both studies suffered limitations from retrospective design, reliance on informants reports for crash histories, and lack of data regarding the nature of driving exposure. Tuokko et al. (1995) examined driving records (insurance claims) of 165 drivers with dementia and found that they had approximately 2.5 times the crash rate of their matched control sample. In contrast, in a study using state records, road crash and violation rates among AD patients did not differ significantly from those of matched controls (Trobe et al., 1996). However, this study did not control for mileage driven, and reduced driving exposure of AD patients may have kept their crash rate equal to that of control subjects. More recently, Carr et al. (2000) reported that a sample of 63 drivers with very mild or mild Clinical Dementia Rating (CDR), showed no difference in state recorded crash rate for the previous 5 year period, when compared to non-demented, older control drivers, even after adjusting for exposure. Carr et al. (2000) note that the drivers with dementia in their study may have been only mildly impaired in their driving skills, with little, if any, impairment in driving skills evident in the preceding 5-year period.

A study of neuropathological findings in 98 older drivers killed in traffic accidents showed that 33% had neuritic plaque scores indicating certain AD, and in a further 20%, findings were suggestive of AD (Johansson et al., 1997). This finding raises the possibility that more accidents are attributable to AD than previously thought. With regard to the reluctance of some AD patients to cease driving, one survey found that 73.7% of Aged Care Assessment Teams had been confronted by the issue of clients that had been judged unsafe to drive, continuing to drive against advice (Fox et al., 1996).

It has been recommended that limitation of driving privileges should be based on demonstration of impaired driving competence, rather than on a clinical diagnosis such as AD (Drachman, 1988; Dobbs, 1997; Carr et al., 2000). Drachman's (1988) objection to excluding people diagnosed with AD from driving is premised on the possibility of minimal functional decline in early AD. He also suggests that the likelihood of loss of driving privileges may result in many people with mild or potentially treatable cognitive impairments refraining from seeking medical advice about continuing to drive. O'Neill (1992) points out that the studies such as that of Friedland et al. (1988) and Lucas-Blaustein et al. (1988) show that a substantial minority of patients with AD, at the time of driving assessment, had suffered no deterioration in driving skills, thus supporting the view that a diagnosis of AD alone is not sufficient to preclude driving. Moreover, there may be considerable variation in the rate of disease progression and nature of disease manifestation in AD, particularly in the earlier stages, and therefore using a diagnosis of AD as a basis for a decision regarding driving is not recommended (Haxby et al., 1992). Hence, given the increasing number of older drivers, the incidence of AD in the elderly and the crash risk for older drivers with AD, it is evident that there is a growing need for procedures for identification of drivers at risk and assessment of driving competence skill for drivers with AD.

ASSESSMENT

Three main approaches to assessing driving competence for AD drivers are described in the literature: off-road techniques, driving simulators, and on-road driving tests. Studies discussed below have examined subjects with AD and other forms of dementia, or have examined groups of older drivers.

OFF-ROAD ASSESSMENT

Mini Mental Status Examination

The Mini Mental Status Examination (MMSE; Folstein et al., 1975) has been frequently used as a measure of severity of dementia as part of an assessment of driving competence, either alone or as part of a neuropsychological test battery (Lucas-Blaustein et al., 1988; Gilley et al., 1991; Logsdon et al., 1992; Hunt et al., 1993; Odenheimer et al., 1994; Fitten et al., 1995). Cessation of driving has been associated with lower MMSE scores (Lucas-Blaustein et al., 1988; Dubinsky et al., 1992; Logsdon et al., 1992), although the MMSE did not distinguish those AD patients who had crashes from those who had not in retrospective crash rate audits (Friedland, 1988; Lucas-Blaustein et al., 1988; Gilley et al., 1991). A mental status exam was found to be a significant predictor of accidents, particularly of intersection accidents, in a group of older drivers (mean age = 70, range 57–83 years) (Ball & Owsley, 1991). Odenheimer et al. (1994) reported a strong correlation between MMSE and driving performance in a group of 30 elderly drivers, of whom six were diagnosed with dementia. However, a large overlap in range of MMSE scores over the global rating of driving performance, which was scored either as pass or fail was observed. Because of this poor correspondence, Odenheimer et al. suggested that MMSE alone was not adequate for predicting driving performance. Fitten et al. (1995) examined the correspondence between performance on several cognitive tasks and a road test. Subjects included two mild dementia groups. They noted limitations for the MMSE's discriminating power. At the upper end of the MMSE range, the MMSE score did not correlate with the drive score, suggesting limited usefulness of this test as a driver screening device. In summary, the MMSE has not been found useful for identifying on individual basis those with dementia who are likely to experience difficulty with driving, because of insufficient sensitivity and specificity.

Cognitive Tasks

The relationship between performance on cognitive tasks or neuropsychological measures and driving for people with dementia has been investigated in several studies (Kapust & Weintraub, 1992; Hunt et al., 1993; Odenheimer et al., 1994; Fitten et al., 1995; Fox et al., 1997). Interestingly, a UK study in 2001 noted that out of 92 psychologists in neuropsychological settings, 70% reported that they use neuropsychological tests to make recommendations regarding fitness to drive; however, 51% are not confident about this (Christie et al., 2001).

In a pilot project where two AD patients underwent neurological, neuropsychological and on-road driving evaluation, both patients demonstrated mild to moderate cognitive impairment, but one of the patients was deemed safe to drive in the on-road test while the other was not (Kapust & Weintraub, 1992). In another study the driving ability of 12 subjects with very mild AD, 13 subjects with mild AD, and 13 healthy elderly controls was measured by an on-road test (Hunt et al., 1993). Five (40%) of the mild AD subjects had sufficient impairment to be judged to have failed the on-road test, while all other subjects were judged to have passed the test. In this study, neither subject self-assessment nor caregiver perceptions of driving ability consistently predicted driving performance (Hunt et al., 1993). Attention, language, and visuoperceptual abilities were found to be correlated with driving performance although the on-road test in this study was only partly standardized. Hunt et al. concluded that performance-based road test evaluations are necessary to determine driving skills, although they also suggested that cognitive screening measures should be further developed to predict driving ability in AD.

Fitten et al. (1995) examined road driving ability and performance on attention, perception, and memory tasks in five groups of drivers: two mild dementia groups and three control groups. The best predictors of the drive score were the Sternberg Memory Test, MMSE, and visual tracking performance. In another study, medical and neuropsychological examination of subjects with a diagnosis of probable AD who were still actively driving was followed by a standardized road driving test (Fox et al., 1997). None of the neuropsychology test scores were associated significantly with the result of the on-road test. Bieliauskas et al. (1998) examined the performance of nine subjects with dementia of the Alzheimer type (DAT) and nine age-matched controls, on neuropsychological testing and an on-road driving test. None of the neuropsychological tests correlated significantly with driving errors for controls, and only Shipley Institute of Living Scale scores and Southern California Figure-Ground Test scores showed significant correlations with driving errors in subjects with DAT. They concluded that neuropsychological tests showed relatively weak overall power in predicting measured driving errors and suggested that neuropsychological test measures may be more predictive of challenge-related driving performance, rather than overlearned skills (Bieliauskas et al., 1998).

An attentional measure termed the Useful Field of View (UFOV) has been investigated with regard to crash frequency in older drivers. The UFOV involves the earliest pre-attentive stage of visual attention and refers to the area of the visual field in which information can be rapidly obtained without eye and head movements (Ball, 1997). The size of the UFOV has been linked to crash frequency, particularly intersection crashes, in older drivers of both good and poor mental status. Ball (1997) noted that within a group of drivers with poor mental state, primarily due to dementia, those individuals with intact UFOV did not crash at a higher rate than age-matched individuals with similarly intact UFOV and good mental state, and concluded that performance-based tests better distinguish crash-free from crash-prone drivers than a diagnosis of dementia.

Duchek et al. (1997, 1998) have further investigated the relationship between specific aspects of visual attention and on-road driving performance, in normal older control subjects, subjects with mild DAT and subjects with very mild DAT. Subjects were administered three visual attention tasks (visual search, visual monitoring, and UFOV), a battery of psychological tests and an on-road driving test. Results indicated that UFOV performance was related to dementia severity, with a reduction in UFOV being associated with increasing dementia severity. UFOV performance was correlated with on-road driving performance. However, it is noteworthy that the UFOV task was very difficult for the mild dementia subjects to perform (only six of 29 subjects were able to complete the task), so that a simpler version of the task would be necessary for screening of subjects with dementia. Driving scores decreased with increasing dementia severity. Of the visual attention measures, overall error rate and reaction time in visual search were the best predictors of the driving test score. Of the psychological test measures, performance on the Boston Naming Test was the only significant predictor of driving. However, visual search performance was more predictive of on-road driving performance than general cognitive status or psychological test performance. Duchek et al. (1997, 1998) concluded that although general cognitive status may be useful for identifying individuals at risk of unsafe driving, measures of selective attention (visual search) may better differentiate safe from unsafe drivers with DAT.

A brief, simply administered Traffic Sign Naming Test, requiring the identification of 10 traffic signs, was reported to successfully distinguish 74% of subjects ($n = 70$) with mild or moderate DAT from normal subjects ($n = 66$) matched for age, sex, education, and socioeconomic status (Cox et al., 1998). Although 11% of the normal subjects were misclassified as demented, Carr and colleagues suggested that the test showed considerable promise for screening purposes of identifying older drivers requiring further assessment of driving skill. A Traffic Sign Recognition test is already required for license renewal in the state of North Carolina (Stutts et al., 1998). A study which included a large sample ($n = 3,238$) of older drivers applying for renewal of their North Carolina driver's license, examined the usefulness of five tests of cognitive function, including a timed Traffic Recognition test, for identifying drivers with elevated crash risk (Stutts et al., 1998). History of crash involvement for the 3-year period prior to testing was available for subjects through state driver history files. Results confirmed previous findings that older drivers with reduced cognitive function are significantly more likely to have been involved in crashes, after controlling for age, race and driving exposure, although the observed effect was relatively small. However, the individual cognitive tests employed in this study were not found to be effective for screening high crash risk drivers (Stutts et al., 1998).

A study involving 407 elderly drivers (aged 62 and above) found significant correlations between unsafe driving incidents in a structured road test, and deficiencies on computerized measures of attentional, perceptual, cognitive, psychomotor, and visual abilities ($r = 0.3 - 0.5$) (McKnight & McKnight, 1999). A total score based on all ability measures correctly identified 80% of incident-involved drivers, while misidentifying 20% of the incident-free drivers. The authors noted that intercorrelations between measured abilities were high, suggesting the need for caution in interpreting reported relationships between individual abilities and unsafe driving incidents. More recently, a study of 84 elderly drivers (aged over 65 years) found that four neuropsychological tests, movement perception, useful field of view, cognitive flexibility and selective attention, could account for 64% of the variance of the total score on the road test (De Raedt & Ponjaert-Kristoffersen, 2000a). However, neuropsychological tests scores could account for only 19% of the variance of self reported at-fault

accidents in the previous year, suggesting that the relationship between performance on cognitive tasks and accident risk may be more complex. Investigating
accident risk may require exploration of capacity for compensation strategies
while driving, a well as identification of driving deficits (De Raedt & Ponjaert-
Kristoffersen, 2000b).

Despite the variable findings, there are some consistent results that have
been reported about the use of cognitive test and driving among individuals
with dementia. The most recent report summarizing this, comes from a meta-
analysis conducted by Reger et al. (2004). The study included 27 primary studies and reported that when studies used control groups a significant relationship
between cognitive measures and on-road and non-road (e.g., simulator) driving measures were significant. However, when studies using a control group
were excluded, more specific findings were identified including moderate correlations between visuospatial skills and on-road and off-road measures, and
between mental status (i.e., MMSE) and non-road tests. The authors concluded
that the findings demonstrate that cognitive/neuropsychological testing makes
a significant contribution to predicting driving ability; however, it does not
indicate at what level of impairment the individual is unfit to drive (Reger
et al., 2004).

In addition to cognition, recent studies have also begun to examine the role of
unawareness of deficit among driving with dementia. It is estimated that 81% of
individuals with AD display anosgnosia, or the unawareness of their impairments
or deficits (Reed et al., 1993). Researchers have also shown that as the severity
of dementia increases, level of awareness decreases (Sevush & Leve, 1993; Ott
et al., 1996). The raised concern is that individuals who are unaware that they
are having difficulty are less likely to stop or limit their own driving in spite of
significant safety hazards. For example, a study conducted by Hunt et al. (1997)
found that 38% of individuals with AD who failed a road test nevertheless considered themselves to be safe drivers. To date, much work has focused on the
cognitive substrates underlying changes in driving ability. Yet, these relationships
do not account for all of the variability in driving performance. Researchers alike
agree that cognitive tests alone are not sensitive and specific enough to determine
driving capacity (Cox et al., 1998). One recent review found that self awareness
of mild changes in sensory and cognitive functioning may lead older adults in
otherwise good health to drive less or to change their driving habits (Kington
et al., 1994). Cotrell and Wild (1999) found results that suggest that awareness
of deficits in attention may lead to appropriate restriction of driving behaviors.
However, even an awareness of attention deficits led to restrictions in only certain driving behaviors (therefore, awareness is modality specific). This was further examined in a study that administered a discrepancy questionnaire (general
awareness), a driving safety questionnaire, a road test, and driving safety evaluation following the road test to individuals with AD and a matched control group
(Wild & Cotrell, 2003). The findings indicated that that a lack of awareness
was positively related to lack of accuracy in self-rated driving skill across the

combined AD and control groups, with an increased correlation when the AD group alone was examined. This present study compared different awareness assessments for driving. They agree that awareness of deficit varies both within patients and between patients. In sum, even if people are aware of their cognitive deficit, they may be unaware of the consequences of these deficits.

Medical Examination

While data increasingly shows risks to individuals and the community associated with driving by people with dementia, there are few guidelines to assist physicians in determining who can or cannot drive, even though physicians are very frequently involved in the determination of driving competence for both the elderly and individuals with dementia. A review in 1993 of North American procedures for driver licensing and medical review reported that 13 jurisdictions require physicians to report potentially dangerous drivers, 11 protect the physician by law from legal action by the driver, and in 20 jurisdictions the reports are confidential (Poser, 1993). An additional 12 jurisdictions give statutory authorization for physicians to report such drivers but do not require that they do so. Since 1988 physicians in California have been required to report dementia cases to their local health departments, who then forward the information to the Department of Motor Vehicles (DMV).

In the United Kingdom the relevant act requires notification to the licensing authority by the license holder (i.e., the patient) of diagnosis of a disability likely to affect safe driving, frequently after advice from a physician (King et al., 1992). In Australia, national uniform guidelines for health professionals on assessing fitness to drive and associated legal obligations have been approved by all Australian driver licensing authorities. Under national uniform driver licensing laws, any person reporting a driver to the relevant authority in good faith because of doubt about a driver's fitness to drive, will be protected from civil and criminal liability throughout Australia.

Reuben (1993) has suggested that scientific evidence is lacking to support a physician's examination as a means of correctly identifying safe older drivers. Review of the literature revealed little attention to the investigation of the efficacy of medical assessment in correctly distinguishing safe from unsafe drivers with dementia, even though in most countries this task legally remains a responsibility of physicians. Therefore, while many physicians have legal responsibility for assessing the safety of their patients to drive, there is a lack of information to assist them in this process. One study investigated the relationship between a medical examination and an on-road driving test in a group of drivers with AD ($n = 19$) (Fox et al., 1997). No relationship was observed neither between any of the medical variables and the global judgement of driving competence, nor between the physician's prediction of driving test outcome and the final rating of driving competence. The authors suggested that the lack of an association may be attributable to the low frequency of abnormal medical variables, and concluded that reliance on medical evaluation alone to determine fitness to drive may not be justified except in those instances where medical factors impact on driving, such as visual field defect (Fox et al., 1997). Comorbidity is an important issue, particularly in the case of elderly drivers, for whom cognitive dysfunction may co-occur with motor or visual dysfunction, for example, potentially resulting in cumulatively higher risks for safe driving. Fitten (1997) noted that for the physician, early or mild dementia poses a difficult problem of detection and reporting with ethical and legal ramifications, and suggested the development of a screening protocol for disease-related cognitive impairment, with positive cases being reported to the relevant authorities for further processing.

In 2000, the American Academy of Neurology published a practice parameter regarding AD and driving (Dubinsky et al., 2000). Two recommendations were made. Firstly, drivers with AD whose Clinical Dementia Rating (CDR) is 1 or greater should not drive, because of driving performance errors and a substantially increased accident rate. Secondly, drivers with possible AD with a severity of CDR 0.5 should be considered for referral for driving performance evaluation. Furthermore, because of the high likelihood of disease progression, reassessment of dementia severity and of appropriateness of continued driving every 6 months was recommended. This follow-up recommendation was evaluated in a prospective longitudinal study of 58 healthy control, 21 individuals with very mild AD, and 29 individuals with mild AD. In this study participants underwent a standardized on-road test approximately every 6 months for a 3-year period. Analysis of the survival curves generated for each group supported the recommendation to conduct driver evaluation every 6 months for persons with very mild and mild dementia of the Alzheimer's type (Duchek et al., 2003). A more recent systematic review that focused on providing evidence for the optimal frequency of follow-up (Molnar et al., 2006) reviewed 164 articles on dementia and driving, of which only 16 met their inclusion/exclusion criteria. Of these only three studies includedrecommendations of specific periods of follow-up. The authors conclude that additional longitudinal studies were needed and that until then, data describing the progression of AD can help guide recommendations.

While these studies serve to provide clinicians with some guidelines, potential difficulties with implementation of these parameters have been noted. For example, the AD patient or their family may not accept the physician's recommendation for discontinuation of driving. Additionally, appropriately qualified driving examiners may not be available in many locations, particularly outside of urban areas, and the cost of such driving examinations may be prohibitive for some patients (Foley et al., 2001).

Thus while physicians have a significant responsibility for determining "medical" competence to drive, in practice such a clinical decision is difficult because of lack of standards and effective guidelines. Moreover, as the actual driving situation is complex and constantly changing, the validity of isolated physiological testing is questionable with regard to safe driving (Reuben et al., 1988).

DRIVING SIMULATORS

With the increasing number of advanced, interactive and affordable driving simulation options, the number of studies that have examined performance on driving simulators by subjects with AD or other dementias has also increased in recent years. As such, the findings from these studies are heavily dependent on the type of driving simulator that is employed. Commercial driving simulators generally are not interactive, so that the stimulus material presented to the subject does not change in reaction to the subject's response or lack of response, resulting in a lack of face validity for many subjects. Performance on commercial driving simulators has not been found to be significantly associated with on-road driving ability in drivers with brain impairment (Galski et al., 1992; Hopewell & Price). More recently, interactive driving simulators have been developed which are more realistic and can be programmed to present a variety of traffic situations (Brouwer & Van Zomeren, 1992; Reinach et al., 1997; Cox et al., 1998; Cox et al., 1999; Rizzo et al., 2001).

Performance on a commercial driving simulator, MMSE and two measures of functional status, Katz-ADL (activities of daily living) and Lawton-IADL (instrumental activities of daily living), was investigated in a study with 41 subjects with probable AD (Shua-Haim & Gross, 1996). Results showed that for MMSE scores of less than 23, a significantly greater proportion of subjects failed the driving simulator assessment, relative to MMSE scores of greater than 23. No correlation was found between scores obtained on either the ADL or IADL and the driving-simulator task. The authors concluded that people obtaining a MMSE score of 22 or less should undergo an on-road driving evaluation, and furthermore commented that the validity of the driving simulator had not been tested (Shua-Haim & Gross, 1996). Another study utilized an interactive driving simulator and produced crash plots for collision avoidance scenarios presented to a single subject, an 80-year old male diagnosed with AD, who had been involved in two at-fault crashes in the previous 3 years (Reinach et al., 1997). Crash plots were produced by analysis of vehicle speed, path, steering wheel position, pedal positions and driver gaze, up to the moment of simulated impact. Several types of antecedent errors were noted, ranging from responding inappropriately with controls to not responding at all. The crashes in the simulator paralleled the subject's crash history on the road. The interactive driving simulator therefore permitted direct observation of driver-safety errors, with no risk of injury to the driver or the observer.

More recently, 18 drivers with dementia and 12 elderly non-demented control drivers drove an interactive simulator on a virtual highway in a scenario where the approach to an intersection triggered the illegal entry of another vehicle into the intersection. To avoid collision, the driver had to perceive, attend to, and interpret the roadway situation, formulate an evasive plan, and then exert appropriate action on the accelerator, brake or steering controls, all under pressure of time (Rizzo et al., 2001). Results showed that 6 of 18 drivers with AD (33%) experienced crashes in the simulator, while none of the control drivers did. It was noteworthy that none of the drivers in this study committed a safety error while driving on the simulated highway preceding the intersection incursion. The authors comment that unless an experimental driving task poses sufficient challenge, the likelihood of observing meaningful safety errors for predicting driver fitness is low (Rizzo et al., 2001).

More recently, researchers examined the relationship between performance on neuropsychological test and performance on a driving simulator Szlyk et al. (2002). The researchers generated a battery of 12 neuropsychological measures based on feedback from an extensive survey of practicing neuropsychologist. This was followed by administration of these tests, along with a driving simulation to 22 licensed drivers between the ages of 67 and 91. Participants were catagorized into a control group or a suspected dementia group based on MMSE scores. The findings indicated difference between the group indicating that drivers with suspected dementia drove significantly slower and had problems with lane boundary crossing.

The predictive validity of such interactive simulator assessment has not yet been demonstrated and may be difficult to determine, without allowing individuals thought to be at high risk of crashing to continue to drive and possibly crash. Cox et al. (1999) investigated whether driving performance on an interactive driving simulator predicted occurrence of future accidents among older drivers. Drivers had previously been rated as Low risk or High risk of future accidents on the basis of score on a driving-simulation task. From self-report data, the drivers predicted as being High risk reported having 47 crashes per 1,000,000 miles driven, whereas the Low risk drivers reported six crashes per 1,000,000 miles driven ($p = 0.04$). As driving simulators continue to evolve, improvements in predictability can be realistically anticipated. Further investigation of predictability of driving simulator assessment for both on-road driving ability and crash risk is recommended.

ON-ROAD DRIVING ASSESSMENT

Although on-road driving performance has frequently been adopted as the "gold standard" for driving skill for drivers with dementia, few studies have addressed the validity or reliability of the on-road driving test. Many of the studies have included a small sample size, often because of difficulty in recruitment of drivers with dementia, who may fear possible loss of their license.

In one such study with elderly subjects, some of whom were diagnosed with dementia, a road test featuring a fixed route and use of the same vehicle, conducted at a prescribed time of day in clear weather, was developed by Odenheimer et al. (1994). There were 68 scored tasks in the in-traffic section, including turns, merges, responses to traffic signs and signals, driving straight, and performing more complex manoeuvres such as a three-point turn. To pass a task, all relevant behaviors for that task had to be correctly completed. The behaviors included scanning of the environment, positioning of the vehicle, speed, and use of turn signals. Driving instructions were presented to subjects as single step commands, and subjects were not asked to find their way. This test appeared to rely on operational aspects of driving in determining competence. Reliability and validity of this test were discussed in terms of relationships between the in-traffic scores and a driving instructor's global evaluation of performance ($r = 0.74$, $p < 0.01$), and between averaged road test scores and cognitive measures. The authors noted that while widely accepted by licensing agencies, their criterion standard of a global evaluation by a driving instructor lacked specific information about driving performance.

In another example of a standardized test, a road assessment was conducted on a hospital campus road network on Saturday mornings only, to ensure consistent low level traffic conditions (Fitten et al., 1995). Subjects in this study included two mild dementia groups and three control groups. The road test consisted of a six stage driving course, 2.7 miles long, with each stage presenting a different degree of driving complexity. Every test drive was recorded by a wide-angle camera mounted on the roof of the vehicle above the driver's head. Driving performance was scored by a driving instructor, with a maximum number of points possible for an error free drive. Approximately 80% of the points related to specific actions at each of the six stages, while 20% involved more general aspects of the drive, such as adequate judgement on the road, and lack of direct instructor intervention. Interestingly, as part of their examination of validity of their on-road test, Fitten et al. obtained collision and moving violation records for all older participants, for the 2-year period before their involvement in the study. A negative non-significant correlation was observed between the drive score and number of collisions/moving violations per thousand miles driven.

Hunt et al. (1997a) developed a standardized on-road driving test, and examined interrater reliability and test-retest reliability of the driving test for DAT subjects ($n = 36$ very mild, $n = 29$ mild severity) and age-matched healthy controls ($n = 58$). Their test was developed to include driving behaviors associated with higher rates of motor vehicle crashes in the elderly, such as negotiating intersections. A standardized route providing a variety of road and traffic situations was used. Test-retest reliability was assessed by having a subset of subjects return for a road test 1 month after their initial road test. Two measures were derived from the driving test: a global rating (safe, marginal or unsafe as determined independently by the driving instructor and the study investigator), and a quantitative score (three-point scale scored for specific manoeuvres at pre-specified locations by the study investigator). A significant association between global rating of driving performance and dementia severity rating was reported. The quantitative scores were categorized, and each category was found to be correlated significantly with the global rating. Interrater reliability was reported as 0.85 for the driving instructor and study investigator, and as 0.96 for the three study investigators. With regard to test-retest reliability, reliability of the global rating by the driving instructor was 0.53, and for the quantitative score reliability was 0.76. The group of drivers rated as "marginal" on the global rating of driving performance contributed disproportionately to the relatively low test-retest stability of the global rating.

Hunt et al. (1997a) concluded that dementia adversely affects driving performance even in the mild stage of severity, although some individuals with DAT seem to drive safely for some time after disease onset. Approximately half of the subjects eligible declined to participate in this study, possibly because they were concerned about their driving ability. A higher proportion of subjects may have been rated as unsafe if all eligible subjects, including those worried about their driving, had participated. The authors suggested that the lower test-retest reliability for the global rating may be due to variability in driving performance across testing sessions. On the basis of qualitative observations of driving and caregiver reports, Hunt et al. also suggested that drivers with cognitive impairment seek the actions of other drivers to follow the flow of traffic, such as mimicking preceding drivers, so that presence of environmental cues, such as other vehicles, may affect driving performance from one occasion to the next (Hunt et al., 1997b).

Another study examined the driving performance of 19 subjects with probable AD on a standardized open road driving evaluation (Fox et al., 1997). The outcome measure was the joint rating by two observers of overall driving competence, as either pass or fail. Additionally, one observer scored each driving manoeuvre, and a correct driving actions score was calculated. As all subjects except one were still driving and all wished to continue to drive, it is noteworthy that 12 subjects were judged to have failed the driving evaluation, while the remaining 7 were judged to have passed. Duration of the disease was not related to the final result. The on-road test was internally consistent, and the observers rating of overall driving competence was related strongly to the objective score of total correct driving actions. The authors concluded that a diagnosis of AD may not be sufficient criteria for cessation of driving, and recommended instead an objective on-road evaluation for determining driving competence in people with AD, with regular review for those patients with AD who continue to drive (Fox et al., 1997). There are important cost considerations associated with on-road driving evaluations. For some individuals with AD, driving is not a realistic goal because of significant cognitive decline, and driving evaluation may not be necessary nor advisable because of safety concerns. The development of screening protocols to identify such individuals is an important research question that requires further attention.

Dobbs and colleagues (Dobbs, 1997; Dobbs et al., 1998) examined the type of errors committed by older drivers with cognitive decline, predominantly DAT ($n = 155$), and by two control groups consisting of young ($n = 30$) and older ($n = 68$) drivers, on a driving test requiring closed course and open road driving. The open road course consisted of 37 driving manoeuvres, emphasizing those manoeuvres implicated in the crashes of older drivers. Driving errors were scored with a procedure typical of driver licensing tests, and at the conclusion of the drive, the driving evaluator made a global rating of driving performance. A lack of correspondence between the driving error scores and the driving evaluators rating of driving was noted, and was attributed to the number of driving errors committed that are typical of experienced drivers, and not indicative of declining competence. This finding is in contrast to the association between the expert judgement of driving performance and the objective correct driving actions score reported by Fox et al. (1997). Fox et al. scored correct driving actions for each part of a driving manoeuvre, whereas Dobbs et al. scored demerit points for driving errors, as is customary for many driver license tests. The positive versus negative scoring and variance in the unit of driving behavior being observed may at least partially account for the difference in association between objective scores and expert judgements in these studies.

Analysis of the driving errors in the Dobbs study (Dobbs et al., 1998) showed that one set of errors, "hazardous", was made almost exclusively by subjects from the dementia group, and differentiated cognitively impaired drivers from normal drivers. Half of the hazardous errors occurred when the vehicle was changing lanes, merging, or approaching intersections. A second set of errors discriminated amongst the groups on the basis of frequency and severity, with the least number of errors committed by the young control group and the most frequent by the cognitively impaired group. Such errors included turn positioning, minor positioning, and overcautiousness. A final set of errors were made equally often by all subject groups. While this final group of errors might result in failure of a driver licensing test, they were considered as "bad habit" errors, and were not indicative of a decline in driving competence. Dobbs et al. (1998) concluded that the typical license test procedure is unsuitable for the task of distinguishing safe from unsafe experienced older drivers. They further argued for the development of an empirically based scoring scheme for assessment of driving performance of individuals with dementia instead of the use of expert judges or raters to determine fitness to drive, on the basis of the rarity of driving evaluators expert in older drivers, and the potential lack of consistency between evaluation centers.

OTHER DEMENTIAS

Other less frequently occurring dementias include illnesses such as Parkinson's Disease (PD) and Huntington's Disease (HD). Diagnostic medical confirmation, neuropsychological assessment, and the risk management of such disorders should be similar to the strategies employed for Senile Dementia of the Alzheimer type.

Parkinson's Disease

This common disease, known since ancient times, was first clinically described by James Parkinson (1817). The disease generally begins between 40 and 70 years of age, with the peak age of onset in the sixth decade. It is infrequent before 30 years of age, and most series contain a somewhat larger proportion of men. The core syndrome is one of expressionless face, poverty and slowness of voluntary movement, "resting" tremor, stooped posture, axial instability, rigidity, and festinating gait. Although most are familiar with the motor effects of the disease, cognitive decline may also be seen. Patients therefore experience not only a progressive loss of motor control, but eventually are at risk for cognitive and emotional deterioration. Cognitive symptoms are also mostly subcortical, and include slowed information processing, executive impairment, memory loss, and associated personality changes.

In regards to driving, earlier work identified a significant accident risk among individuals with PD (Borromei et al., 1999). More recently, research with this population has focused on specific difficulties, including a study that examined the ability for visual search and recognition of roadside targets and safety errors during a landmark and traffic sign identification task. The researchers examined 79 drivers with PD and 151 neurologically normal older adults. All participants underwent a battery of visual, cognitive, and motor tests and an experimental drive in a simulator that required them to report sightings of specific landmarks and traffic signs along a four-lane commercial strip. The findings indicated that drivers with PD identified significantly fewer landmarks and traffic signs, and they committed more at-fault safety errors during the task than control subjects, even after adjusting for baseline errors (Uc et al., 2006).

A more recent UK study examined driving ability of 154 individuals with PD referred to a driving assessment center where a combination of clinical tests, reaction times on a test rig and an in-car driving test were used (Singh et al., 2006). They report that the majority of cases (104, 66%) were able to continue driving although 46 individuals required an automatic transmission and 10 others needed car modifications. Physical disease severity, age, presence of other associated medical conditions particularly dementia, duration of disease, brake reaction time on a test rig and score on a driving test (all $p < 0.0001$) predicted the ability to drive. The authors noted that the most important features in distinguishing safety to drive in their sample were severity of physical disease, reaction time, moderate disease associated with another medical condition and high score on car testing (Singh et al., 2007).

In sum, some of the significant cognitive factors identified as relevant to driving also are important in drivers with PD. However, given the additional motor deficits associated with this disorder and the progressiveness of the disease, monitoring of symptoms and repeated evaluations are warranted among this clinical population.

Huntington's Disease

This disease, distinguished by the triad of dominant inheritance, choreoathetosis, and dementia, derives its eponym from George Huntington (1872). Although relatively rare, in university hospital centers this is one of the most frequently observed types of hereditary nervous system disease. The usual age of onset is in the fourth and fifth decades, but 3–5% begin before the 15th year and some even in childhood. In 28% of cases, symptoms become apparent after 50 years. The progression of the disease is slower in older patients. Once begun, the disease progresses relentlessly.

The mental disorders associated with HD assumes several subtle forms long before the deterioration of cognitive functions becomes evident. In approximately half the cases, slight and often annoying alterations of character are the first to appear. Patients begin to find fault with everything, they may be suspicious, irritable, impulsive, eccentric, untidy, or excessively religious, or they may exhibit a false sense of superiority. Poor self-control may be reflected in outbursts of temper, fits of despondency, alcoholism, or sexual promiscuity. Disturbances of mood, particularly depression, are common and may constitute the most prominent symptoms early in the disease.

Eventually other cognitive functions deteriorate and the patient becomes less communicative and more socially withdrawn. Diminished work performance, inability to manage household responsibilities, disturbances of sleep, difficulty in maintaining attention, impaired concentration, deficits in learning new material, and mental rigidity become apparent, along with loss of fine manual skills. Since remote memory is relatively spared, such a gradual deterioration of intellectual function has been characterized as a "subcortical dementia." Increased deterioration of motor functions and chorea (a relatively ceaseless occurrence of a wide variety of rapid, highly complex, jerky movements which appear to be coordinated but are in fact involuntary) usually follow.

Rebok et al. (1995) assessed the influence of the neurological and cognitive impairments of HD on automobile driving. These authors found that HD patients performed significantly worse than control subjects on the driving-simulator tasks and were more likely to have been involved in a collision in the preceding 2 years (58% of HD versus 11% of control subjects). Patients with collisions were less functionally impaired but had slower simple reaction time scores than did those without collisions. Presumably all such patients will eventually cease driving in one way or another as this terminal disease progresses.

PUBLIC POLICY ISSUES

Public policy issues have concerned the development of procedures to identify, screen, and regulate those drivers with dementia who are at higher risk of crashes (Eberhard, 1997). The state of California has since 1988 required physicians to report persons with dementia to their local health department, who then forward the information to the DMV. The DMV in California subsequently revised its policies regarding drivers with dementia (Reuben & St George, 1996). A new physician completed driver medical evaluation form for dementia and a new reporting form for non-physicians were created, along with a new schema for evaluating drivers with dementia. The medical evaluation form required physicians to rate specific cognitive and behavioral disturbances and to provide an assessment of overall degree of impairment. Definitions of mild, moderate, and severe impairment were provided. In cases where a physician's initial report indicated that dementia severity was moderate or advanced, the drivers license was revoked immediately. For early or mild dementia, the driver was scheduled for reexamination by the DMV, entailing a standard knowledge test, an interview with a driver-safety hearing officer, a vision test, and a special driving test. Failure of any of these tests, except the vision test, automatically resulted in license cancellation. The special driving test is longer than standard license tests and requires a specific set of road instructions, but is not any more difficult than the license test. If a driver with dementia passes all of these tests, they are scheduled for review in 6 to 12 months. This procedure does not require DMV staff to make judgements about medical competence to drive, but instead to base their judgements on the driver's performance on the evaluations. It is noteworthy that since the introduction of the 1988 rules, the incidence of reporting of drivers with dementia has been lower than anticipated, possibly because of concerns that reporting a patient may jeopardize the patient–doctor relationship (Reuben & St George, 1996). The impact of the reporting requirements and subsequent restrictions on licenses have not been evaluated yet.

More recently, the California DMV and the National Highway Traffic Safety Administration commenced work on development of a licensing agency assessment battery for elderly drivers with dementia or other medical conditions (Janke & Eberhard, 1998). Existent license renewal procedures were considered inadequate for determining whether older applicants were safe and competent drivers. One of the goals of the research was to provide a basis for a graded licensing system, in which drivers not fit to drive unrestrictedly would be given advisory or mandatory restrictions to limit the conditions of their driving. The drivers under study had been referred for reexamination because of various impairing conditions. Reexamination is not part of the normal license renewal process and involves only a small percentage of drivers. A three-tier system was proposed, with the first tier consisting of brief screening tests, and the second tier requiring longer tests for those who performed poorly on the first tier, and also those referred by physicians, family members, etc. The third tier was a road test. Subjects were 75 drivers referred for reexamination and 31 paid volunteers. Within the first tier tests, measures found useful for detecting impairment in this sample included number of observable disabilities, low contrast acuity test errors and performance on an automatized version of the Trail Making Test. The authors suggested that with the addition of a few simple tests, renewal applicants identified as having impaired functioning could then go on to receive counselling about their driving or restricted licenses, be referred for further health assessment, or be examined in more detail on driving-related skills. With regard to second tier tests, some tasks, including a driving-simulator task and a static visual acuity time score, were found to be predictive of weighted errors on one of the road driving tests.

Waller (1988) has argued for several modifications to the process of renewal licensing of older drivers. These include an increase in the frequency of routine reexaminations for the purpose of license renewal after the age of 75 years, along with a graduated driving reduction program, which would gradually reduce the amount and kinds of driving done so that the elderly would be slowly removed from the driving population as their performance became less proficient. Vision testing should be expanded to include visual acuity under reduced illumination and dynamic visual acuity. It was also recommended that states create an advisory board for licensing of elderly drivers. Ensuring the provision of counselling services for driving alternatives would be one important function of such an advisory board.

Another good state model currently in effect is that of the Maine Functional Abilities Profiles (1985). Maine was the first of the United States to devise a functional impairment rating system for her disabled drivers. Maine has also made provision that the reporting of an impaired driver by a physician, psychologist, or "other person ... in good faith shall have immunity for any damages claimed as a result of so doing" (29 M.R.S.A. SS 51, 547, 581, 2241, and 2241-A). The state has also added a physician to its medical advisory board, though a psychologist has yet to be added.

CONCLUSION

The absence of consistency in findings of studies examining driving performance of subjects with dementia is not surprising, as the outcome measures employed vary considerably. In the studies described above, outcome measures have included retrospective crash rates, subsequent crash rates, informants reports, driving simulator performance, and open road driving tests. Despite the variability in methodologies, several groups have reported that patients with dementia who drive have a higher risk of crashes, when reduced mileage is accounted for (Friedland, 1988; Lucas-Blaustein et al., 1988; Tuokko et al., 1995). Nonetheless, some individuals with dementia have been judged safe to drive on the basis of a road test, at least in the early stages of the disease, and therefore a diagnosis of dementia alone is not sufficient to preclude driving on an individual basis (Hunt et al., 1993; Fox et al., 1997). Instead, a means of identification of drivers with dementia who are at risk of crashes and who are no longer competent to drive is required. Several investigators have concluded that for examination of drivers with dementia, competence-based tests are required which are fair, cost-effective, and appropriate for experienced older drivers (Fox et al., 1997; Dobbs et al., 1998). An appropriate test is one that is standardized, distinguishes "bad habit" driving errors from dangerous driving errors, and includes some complex traffic situations, while simultaneously not discriminating against the older driver. There is evidence that current driver license type tests are not appropriate for older drivers with dementia as a means of determining driver competence, because of their focus on "bad habit" driving behaviors rather than on dangerous driving behaviors. Studies of on-road driving behavior of patients with dementia indicate that older drivers with a range of cognitive abilities can be safely and reliably evaluated by a road test, with validity equal to that of driver license tests.

However, given the large cost implications and service provision requirements for on-road testing of all drivers with dementia, the development of a screening protocol is urgently required, to identify drivers at risk. Subsequently, positive cases could then undergo further assessment. Studies reviewed suggest that screening procedures for drivers with dementia could include visual attention measures such as UFOV (Ball, 1997), visual search tasks (Duchek et al., 1998), and a Traffic Sign Naming Test (Carr et al., 1998). Screening could be conducted by licensing agencies at time of license renewal, or by physicians or other health professionals. Screening by licensing agencies might be more effective if the time period between license renewals was decreased, particularly for older drivers (Waller, 1988). Ideally, drivers who perform poorly on the screening protocol could then be referred for assessment of actual driving behavior during an on-road driving test. Further development of interactive driving simulators might allow assessment of driving abilities in an off-road setting, with no risk to the driver or other road users. However, before performance on interactive driving simulators can be used as evidence of unsafe driving, with implications for license revocation, further research to examine the predictive validity of simulator driving for on-road driving is required.

Which agency should perform the on-road driving assessment is unclear. It is likely that driver license agencies will not have sufficient resources to complete large numbers of on-road driving tests. With regard to an on-road driving test for drivers with dementia, the occurrence of hazardous errors has been found to discriminate between impaired drivers and age-matched controls (Dobbs et al., 1998). Other useful information for identifying drivers at risk which could be requested from family members includes any incidences of getting lost, perplexity while driving, and requiring prompts from passengers. Introducing restrictions on driving, such as not driving at night or driving only within a certain radius of home, has been suggested as a means of implementing a graduated driving reduction program. However, one problem with this approach is that there is no evidence that drivers with dementia are any safer driving near their home, for example, or when driving on familiar roads. Regular review of drivers with dementia is essential. Six months has been suggested as an appropriate time interval, unless an increase in disease severity indicates the need for an earlier review. If assessment demonstrates that driving should be ceased, the patient and family should be involved in discussion of transport alternatives including assistance from family and friends, and community transport options so that activities can be continued. Provision of counselling about lifestyle changes and future planning of transportation may be critical to compliance as well as to psychological wellbeing, as driving cessation may be associated with depressive symptoms.

REFERENCES

Ball, K. (1997). Attentional problems and older drivers. *Alzheimer Dis. Assoc. Disord.*, *11*(Suppl. 1), 42–47.

Ball, K., & Owsley, C. (1991). Identifying correlates of accident involvement for the older driver. *Hum. Factors*, *33*(5), 583–595.

Ball, K., Owsley, C., Stalvey, B., Roenker, D. L., Sloane, M. E., & Graves, M. (1998). Driving avoidance and functional impairment in older drivers. *Accid. Anal. Prev.*, *30*(3), 313–322.

Bieliauskas, L. A., Roper, B. R., Trobe, J., Green, P., & Lacy, M. (1998). Cognitive measures, driving safety, and Alzheimer's disease. *Clin. Neuropsych.*, *12*(2), 206–212.

Borromei, A., Caramelli, R., Chieregatti, G., d'Orsi, U., Guerra, L., Lozito, A., & Vargiu, B. (1999). Ability and fitness to drive of parkinson disease patients. *Func. Neurol. New Trends Adap. Behav. Disord. 14*(4), 227–234.

Brouwer, W., & Van Zomeren, E. (1992). Evaluation of driving in traumatically brain-injured persons. *Presentation given at the Second International Congress on Objective Evaluation in Rehabilitation Medicine*, Montreal, October 5–6.

Carr, D. B., Duchek, J., & Morris, J. C. (2000). Characteristics of motor vehicle crashes of drivers with dementia of the Alzheimer type. *J. Am. Geriatr. Soc., 48*, 18–22.

Carr, D. B., LaBarge, E., Dunnigan, K., & Storandt, M. (1998). Differentiating drivers with dementia of the Alzheimer's type from healthy older persons with a traffic sign naming test. *J. Gerontol., 53A*(2), M135–M139.

Christie, N., Savill, T., Buttress, S., Newby, G., & Tyermann, A. (2001). Assessing fitness to drive after head injury: A survey of clinical psychologists. *Neuropsychol. Rehabil., 11*, 45–55.

Cotrell, V., & Wild, K. (1999). Longitudinal study of self-imposed driving restrictions and deficit awareness in patients with Alzheimer disease. *Alzheimer Dis. Assoc. Disord., 13*, 151–156.

Cox, D. J., Quillian, W. C., THorndike, F. P., Kovatchev, B. P., & Hanna, G. (1998). Evaluating driving performance of outpatients with Alzheimer disease. *J. Am. Board Fam. Pract., 11*, 264–271.

Cox, D. J., Taylor, P., & Kovatchev, B. (1999). Driving simulation performance predicts future accidents among older drivers. *J. Am. Geriatr. Soc., 47*, 361–362.

De Raedt, R., & Ponjaert-Kristoffersen, I. (2000a). The relationship between cognitive/neuropsychological factors and car driving performance in older adults. *J. Am. Geriatr. Soc., 48*, 1664–1668.

De Raedt, R., & Ponjaert-Kristoffersen, I. (2000b). Can strategic and tactical compensation reduce crash risk in older drivers? *Age Ageing, 29*, 517–521.

Dobbs, A. R. (1997). Evaluating the driving competence of dementia patients. *Alzheimer Dis. Assoc. Disord., 11*(Suppl. 1), 8–12.

Dobbs, A. R., Heller, R. B., & Schopflocher, D. (1998). A comparative approach to identify unsafe older drivers. *Accid. Anal. Prev., 30*(3), 363–370.

Drachman, D. A. (1988). Who may drive? Who may not? Who shall decide? *Ann. Neurol., 24*, 787–788.

Drachman, D. A., & Swearer, J. M. (1993). Driving and Alzheimer's disease: The risk of crashes. *Neurology, 43*, 2448–2456.

Dubinsky, R. M., Stein, A. C., & Lyons, K. (2000). Practice parameter: Risk of driving and Alzheimer's disease (an evidence-based review). *Neurology, 54*, 2205–2211.

Dubinsky, R. M., Williamson, A., Gray, C. S., & Glatt, S. L. (1992). Driving in Alzheimer's disease. *J. Am. Geriatr. Soc., 40*, 1112–1116.

Duchek, J. M., Carr, D. B., Hunt, L., Roe, C. M., Xiong, C., Shah, K. et al. (2003). Longitudinal driving performance in early-stage dementia of the Alzheimer type. *JAGS, 51*, 1342–1347.

Duchek, J. M., Hunt, L., Ball, K., Buckles, V., & Morris, J. C. (1997). The role of selective attention in driving and dementia of the Alzheimer type. *Alzheimer Dis. Assoc. Disord., 11*(Suppl. 1), 48–56.

Duchek, J. M., Hunt, L., Ball, K., Buckles, V., & Morris, J. C. (1998). Attention and driving performance in Alzheimer's disease. *J. Gerontol., 53B*(2), P130–P141.

Eberhard, J. W. (1997). Safe mobility for people with Alzheimer disease: A commentary. *Alzheimer Dis. Assoc. Disord., 11*(Suppl. 1), 76–77.

Evans, D. A., Funkenstein, H. H., Albert, M. S., Scheer, P. A., Cook, N. R., Chown, M. J. et al. (1989). Prevalence of Alzheimer's disease in a community population of older adults. *JAMA, 262*, 2551–2556.

Fitten, L. J. (1997). The demented driver: The doctor's dilemma. *Alzheimer Dis. Assoc. Disord., 11*(Suppl 1), 57–61.

Fitten, L. J., Perryman, K. M., Wilkinson, C. J., Little, R. J., Burns, M. M., Pachana, N. et al. (1995). Alzheimer and vascular dementias and driving. *JAMA, 272*, 1360–1365.

Foley, D., Masaki, K., White, L., Ross, G. W., & Eberhard, J. (2001). Practice parameter: Risk of driving and Alzheimer's disease. *Neurology, 56*, 695.

Folstein, M. F., Folstein, S. E., & McHugh, P. R. (1975). Mini-mental state: A practical method for grading the cognitive state of patients for the clinician. *J. Psychiatr. Res.*, *12*, 189–198.

Fox, G. K., Bowden, S. C., Bashford, G. M., & Smith, D. S. (1997). Alzheimer's disease and driving: Prediction and assessment of driving performance. *J. Am. Geriatr. Soc.*, *45*, 949–953.

Fox, G. K., Withaar, F., & Bashford, G. M. (1996). Dementia and driving: A survey of clinical practice in aged care assessment teams. *Aust. J. Ageing*, *15*(3), 111–114.

Friedland, R. P., Koss, E., Kumar, A., Gaine, S., Metzler, D., Haxby, J. V. et al. (1988). Motor vehicle crashes in dementia of the Alzheimer type. *Ann. Neurol.*, *24*, 782–786.

Galski, T., Bruno, R. L., & Ehle, H. T. (1992). Driving after cerebral damage: A model with implications for evaluation. *Am. J. Occ. Th.*, *46*(4), 324–332.

Gilley, D. W., Wilson, R. S., Bennett, D. A., Stebbins, G. T., Bernard, B. A., Whalen, M. E. et al. (1991). Cessation of driving and unsafe motor vehicle operation by dementia patients. *Arch. Intern. Med.*, *151*, 941–946.

Haxby, J. V., Raffaele, K., Gillette, J., Schapiro, M. B., & Rapoport, S. I. (1992). Individual trajectories of cognitive decline in patients with dementia of the Alzheimer type. *JCEN*, *14*(4), 575–592.

Hopewell, C. A, & Price, J. R. (1985). Driving after head injury. *Paper Presentation to the Eighth European Conference of the International Neuropsychological Society*, Copenhagen.

Hunt, L., Morris, J. C., Edwards, D., & Wilson, B. S. (1993). Driving performance in persons with mild senile dementia of the Alzheimer type. *J. Am. Geriatr. Soc.*, *41*, 747–753.

Hunt, L. A., Murphy, C. F., Carr, D., Duchek, J. M., Buckles, V., & Morris, J. C. (1997a). Reliability of the Washington University Road Test. *Arch. Neurol.*, *54*, 707–712.

Hunt, L. A., Murphy, C. F., Carr, D., Duchek, J. M., Buckles, V., & Morris, J. C. (1997b). Environment cueing may affect performance on a road test for drivers with dementia of the Alzheimer type. *Alzheimer Dis. Assoc. Disord.*, *11*(Suppl. 1), 13–16.

Janke, M. K., & Eberhard, J. W. (1998). Assessing medically impaired older drivers in a licensing agency setting. *Accid. Anal. Prev.*, *30*(3), 347–361.

Johansson, K., Bogdanovic, H., Kalimo, H., Winblad, B., & Vlitanen, M. (1997). Alzheimer's disease and apolipoprotein E 4 allele in older drivers who died in automobile accidents. *Lancet*, *349*, 1143–1144.

Kapust, L. R., & Weintraub, S. (1992). To drive or not to drive: Preliminary results from road testing of patients with dementia. *J. Geriatr. Psych. Neurol.*, *5*(October–December), 210–216.

King, D., Benbow, S. J., & Barrett, J. A. (1992). The law and medical fitness to drive – A study of doctors' knowledge. *Postgrad. Med. J.*, *68*, 624–628.

Kington, R., Reuban, D., Rogowski, J., & Lillard, L. (1994). Sociodemographic and health factors in driving patterns after 50 years of age. *Am. J. Public Health*, *84*, 1327–1329.

Levy, D. T., Vernick, J. S., & Howard, K. A. (1995). Relationship between driver's licence renewal policies and fatal crashes involving drivers 70 years or older. *JAMA*, *274*, 1026–1030.

Logsdon, R. G., Teri, L., & Larson, E. B. (1992). Driving and Alzheimer's disease. *J. Gen. Intern. Med.*, *7*, 583–588.

Lucas-Blaustein, M. J., Filipp, L., Dungan, C., & Tune, L. (1988). Driving in patients with dementia. *J. Am. Geriatr. Soc.*, *36*, 1087–1091.

McKnight, A. J., & McKnight, A. S. (1999). Multivariate analysis of age-related driver ability and performance deficits. *Accid. Anal. Prev.*, *31*(5), 445–454.

Molnar, FJ., Patel, A., Marshall, SC., Man-Son-Hing, M., & Wilson, K. (2006). Systematic review of the optimal frequency of follow-up in persons with mild dementia who can drive. *Alzheimer Dis. Assoc. Disord.*, *20*(4), 295–297.

Morris, J. C. (1997). Foreword. *Alzheimer Dis. Assoc. Disord.*, *11*(Suppl. 1), 1–2.

Odenheimer, G. L., Beaudet, M., Jette, A. M., Albert, M. S., Grande, L., & Minaker, K. L. (1994). Performance-based driving evaluation of the elderly driver: Safety, reliability, and validity. *J. Gerontol.*, *49*(4), M153–M159.

Ott, B. R., Lafleche, G., Whelihan, W. M., Buongiorno, G. W., Albert, M. S., & Fogel, B. S. (1996). Impaired awareness of deficits in Alzheimer disease. *Alzheimer Dis. Assoc. Disord.*, *10*(2), 68–76.

O'Neill, D. (1992). The doctor's dilemma: The ageing driver and dementia. *Int. J. Geriatr. Psychiatr.*, 7, 297–301.

Poser, C. M. (1993). Automobile driving fitness and neurological impairment. *J. Neuropsychia.*, 5(3), 342–348.

Rebok, G. W., Bylsma, F. W., Keyl, P. M., Brandt, J., & Folstein, S. E. (1995). Automobile driving in Huntington's disease. *Movement Disord.*, 10(6), 778–787.

Reed, B. R., Jagust, W. J., & Coulter, L. (1993). Anosognosia in Alzheimer's disease: Relationships to depression, cognitive function, and cerebral perfusion. *J. Clin. Exp. Neuropsychol.*, 15, 231–244.

Reger, M. A., Welsh, R. K., Watson, G. S., Cholerton, L. D., Baker, L. D., & Craft, S. (2004). The relationship between neuropsychological functioning and driving ability in dementia: A meta-analysis. *Neuropsychology*, 18, 85–93.

Reinach, S. J., Rizzo, M., & McGehee, D. V. (1997). Driving with Alzheimer disease: The anatomy of a crash. *Alzheimer Dis. Assoc. Disord.*, 11(Suppl 1), 21–27.

Reuben, D. B. (1993). Assessment of older drivers. *Clin. Geriatr. Med.*, 9(2), 449–459.

Reuben, D. B., Silliman, R. A., & Traines, M. (1988). The aging driver. Medicine, policy and ethics. *J. Am. Geriatr. Soc.*, 36, 1135–1142.

Reuben, D. B., & St George, P. (1996). Driving and dementia – California's approach to a medical and policy dilemma. *West J. Med.*, 164, 111–121.

Rizzo, M., McGehee, D. V., Dawson, J. D., & Anderson, S. N. (2001). Simulated car crashes at intersections in drivers with Alzheimer disease. *Alzheimer Dis. Assoc. Disord.*, 15, 10–20.

Sevush, S., & Leve, N. (1993). Denial of memory deficit in Alzheimer's disease. *Am. J. Psychiatr.*, 150(5), 748–751.

Shua-Haim, J. R., & Gross, J. S. (1996). A simulated driving evaluation for patients with Alzheimer's disease. *Am. J. Alzheimer Dis.*, 11(3(May/June)), 2–7.

Singh, R., Pentland, B., Hunter, J., & Provan, F. (2007). Parkinson's disease and driving ability. *J. Neurol. Neurosurg, Psychiatr.* 78, 363–366.

Stutts, J. C., Stewart, J. R., & Martell, C. (1998). Cognitive test performance and crash risk in an older driver population. *Accid. Anal. Prev.*, 30(3), 337–346.

Szlyk, J. P., Myers, L., Zhang, Y. X., Wetzel, L., & Shapiro, R. (2002). Development and assessment of a neuropsychological battery to aid in predicting driving performance. *J. Rehabil. Res. Dev.*, 3(4), 483–496.

Trobe, J. D., Waller, P. F., Cook-Flanagan, C. A., Teshima, S. M., & Bieliauskas, L. A. (1996). Crashes and violations among drivers with Alzheimer disease. *Arch. Neurol.*, 53, 411–416.

Tuokko, H., Tallman, K., Beattie, B. L., Cooper, P., & Weir, J. (1995). An examination of driving records in a dementia clinic. *J. Gerontol.*, 50B(3), S173–S181.

Uc, E. Y., Rizzo, M., Anderson, S. W., Sparks, J., Rodnitzky, R. L., & Dawson, J. D. (2006). Impaired visual search in drivers with Parkinson's disease. *Ann. Neurol.*, 60(4), 407–413.

Waller, P. F. (1988). Renewal licensing of older drivers. In: *Committee for the Study on Improving Mobility and Safety for Older Persons. Transportation in an Aging Society* (Vol. 2) (pp. 72–100). Washington, DC: Transportation Research Board.

Wild, K., & Cotrell, V. (2003). Identifying driving impairment in Alzheimer disease: A comparison of self and observer reports versus driving evaluation. *Alzheimer Dis. Assoc. Disord.*, 17, 27–34.

7

DRIVING AND STROKE

MARIA T. SCHULTHEIS AND CASSANDRA FLEKSHER

Cerebral vascular accidents or strokes are the third leading cause of death in the United States. By definition a stroke occurs as a result of blockage or hemorrhage of a blood vessel leading to the brain. The resulting lack of oxygen supply to the brain results in damage that can manifest itself in a variety of physical, cognitive, and behavioral deficits for the individual. Common difficulties can include hemiparegia or paralysis of upper and lower extremities, speech difficulties, visual perception and visuo-spatial difficulties and changes in cognition (e.g., memory, attention, etc.). Not surprisingly, these deficits can have a significant impact on an individual's activities of daily living and overall quality of life.

Given the high value placed on individual transportation in the United States, it is not surprising that many individuals seek to return to driving after experiencing a stroke. In fact, it is estimated that approximately 30–50% of stroke survivors return to driving (Fisk et al., 1997; Heikkilä et al., 1999; Fisk et al., 2002). Yet, it has also been reported that many stroke survivors do not go through any formal evaluation of their driving ability or receive advice before returning to the road. Therefore, the challenge remains in determining how the various sensory-motor and cognitive impairments resulting from stroke may or may not impact the individuals' performance on the road. To date, although no single measurement can be used to definitively calculate an individuals' driving capacity, much has been learned about driving after stroke. This chapter will summarize the current literature examining driving behaviors after resumption of driving and the assessment and retraining of driving skills after stroke.

STROKE AND DRIVING

It is well-documented that stroke can result from different etiologies and can present in significantly varying degrees of severity. As a result stroke is a major cause of disability effecting approximately 500,000 individuals annually (www. americanstrokeassocaition.org). While the highest incidence is reported in older adults, recent work has identified a growing need for younger adults suffering from strokes (e.g., Bjorkdahl & Sunnerhagen, 2007). Given this fact, it is not surprising that stroke survivors (both young and older) find that driving cessation interferes with activities related to independent living (e.g., working) and consider the resumption of driving after stroke, an important step in their recovery. Long-standing evidence supporting this, first came from studies that demonstrated that stroke survivors who did not resume driving participate in fewer social activities and are more likely to be depressed (Legh-Smith et al., 1986). In addition, one study which specifically focused on driving resumption after mild stroke, found that 50% of individuals returned to driving within the first month after experiencing a stroke (Lee et al., 2003); further underscoring the need for early assessment. Indeed, accuracy in measuring driving safety after stroke is crucial to ensuring that individuals who are safe drivers are not prevented from maintaining their independent mode of transportation and to preventing individuals who are unsafe drivers from posing a danger to themselves and others.

Several studies have documented that of those individuals who drive before their stroke, approximately 30–59% return to driving after their stroke (Fisk et al., 1997; Heikkilä et al., 1999). Of those individuals returning behind-the-wheel, almost one-third report high driving exposure, driving 6 to 7 days/week and/or 100 to 200 miles/week (Fisk et al., 1997). However, more recent findings indicate that stroke survivors drive less when compared to a non-stroke cohort (Fisk et al., 2002). Specifically, although no differences in days per week of driving were seen, non-stroke drivers drove to more places, took more trips and drove more miles (Fisk et al., 2002). Drivers who returned to driving also acknowledged difficulties in varying driving situations, such as making left turns, driving on the interstate and driving in heavy traffic. Despite this, the stroke drivers did not differ from the non-stroke drivers in occurrences of self-reported crashes or citations (Fisk et al., 2002). Overall, stroke drivers appear to be self-regulating their driving behaviors and exposure.

RIGHT VERSUS LEFT

One of the most commonly examined areas of stroke research is in evaluating differences in impairment resulting from strokes in the two hemispheres. Several studies have examined the lesion location and the extent of brain damage incurred to better determine the impact of the resulting impairments on driving performance. Cortical damage in the area of the temporoparietal lobe of the right hemisphere often results in impairments in spatial and perceptual abilities, and attentional and visual skills deficits, such as visual neglect. Physically, a right-hemisphere stroke can often lead to paralysis of the left side of the body, known as left hemiplegia. In contrast cortical damage to the left hemisphere often results in language and speech difficulties and paralysis of the right side of the body, known as right hemiplegia. More global cognitive deficits, such as changes in memory and attention, can not be exclusively associated with one or the other hemisphere. In relation to driving difficulties, several studies have indicated poorer performance in individuals who have sustained a right-hemisphere stroke (Quigley & DeLisa, 1983; Korner-Bitensky et al., 2000; Fisk et al., 2002). These researchers have noted the impact of visuo-spatial and perceptual deficits on driving capacity.

While the physical impairments can then lead to problems with motor reaction time, which can be crucial in driving (e.g., hitting the brakes) and safe maneuvering (e.g., steering), in many cases, adaptive driving equipment can be used to minimize the impact of physical limitations. For example, an adaptive spinner knob can be attached to the steering wheel to allow controlled steering with the use of only one hand or a left gas pedal may be used if the individual is unable to use their right foot to gas or brake. In fact, a recent study by Smith-Arena et al. (2006), found that individuals in an acute rehabilitation setting with higher Motricity Index scores and intact visual fields were more likely to pass an in-clinic driver evaluation. The researchers concluded that physicians could safely identify post-stroke patients most appropriate for driver evaluation when mild physical impairments, normal visual fields, and mild cognitive impairments were present. In sum, while physical challenges resulting from stroke can impact driving performance, it is the cognitive and visual impairments that pose a greater challenge for returning to driving.

DRIVING AFTER STROKE: VISION AND VISUAL ATTENTION

Automobile driving is a routinely performed complex activity, with an estimated 90% of the informational input to the driver being visual (Simms, 1985; Mazer, 2001). Indeed, the demands of driving include navigating a vehicle within a visual environment cluttered with distractors which involves the simultaneous use of central and peripheral vision (Ball et al., 1993; Mazer, 2001). While most states have minimum visual requirements for successful licensure, this is typically limited to visual acuity and on occasion, minimal visual fields. In many of these cases, assessment and treatment with an ophthalmologist can help address these deficits. Subsequently, many states allow the use of corrective lenses and in some case bipolar lenses to help individuals compensate for visual acuity deficits (see Appendix A).

What is more commonly seen after stroke and more challenging to evaluate are visual measures that are more cognitively loaded; for example, visual attention, visual processing speed, and visual scanning skills. In addition, survivors of right-hemisphere strokes may also experience left-sided neglect. Stemming from visual field impairments, left-sided neglect causes the survivor of a right-hemisphere stroke to "forget" or "ignore" objects or people on their left side.

One common standardized measure of visual attention in the driving literature is the Useful Field of View (UFOV). UFOV is a computer-administered and computer-scored test of visual attention (UFOV manual). The UFOV has been widely implemented in studies with elderly drivers and these findings indicate a positive association between driving performance and test scores of the UFOV. In addition, evidence supports that retraining using the UFOV is effective in improving visual attention skills in an elderly population. These findings spurred Mazer et al. (2001) to conduct a pilot study to see if the findings could be replicated in a population of stroke survivors. After assessing 52 individuals who had been referred for a driver evaluation, the researchers found overall lower UFOV scores indicative of poor visual attention, with older individuals performing the most poorly. Preliminary findings indicated moderate test–retest reliability of the UFOV an indication that UFOV scores could significantly improve with training (Mazer et al., 2001). A follow-up study by the same group, further examined the effectiveness of visual attention training with the UFOV on driving performance after stroke. The findings, which compared a group of stroke survivors receiving UFOV training and another receiving traditional computerized visuo-perception retraining, found no significant difference between the two groups, indicating that UFOV training was not significantly more beneficial than traditional interventions (Mazer et al., 2003).

Finally, another study examined UFOV performance across non-stroke drivers, stroke drivers, and stroke non-drivers. Similar to Mazer et al. and consistent with neuropsychological findings, all individuals who had suffered a stroke demonstrated poorer UFOV performance when compared to non-stroke drivers (Fisk & Mennemeier, 2006). In addition, non-driving stroke survivors had greater impairment on attentional measures (including the UFOV); leading the researchers to suggest that attentional impairment may be the trigger for driving cessation after stroke (Fisk et al., 2002). Taken together, while these studies lend some support for the use of the UFOV among drivers who have suffered a stroke, a major weakness of this work is the limited evidence that UFOV performance is related to actual driving performance. That is, there are no current studies that have directly examined neither the ecological nor the predictive validity of UFOV performance on a "real world" driving criterion or outcome measure.

Another off-road assessment tool that focuses on visual measures is the Dynavision apparatus, which is manufactured by Performance Enterprises (Ontario, Canada). Specifically, the Dynavision is designed to train visual scanning, peripheral visual awareness, visual attention, and visuo-motor reaction time across a broad, active visual field. It also includes features that require trainees to execute complex visuo-motor response sequences, to use basic cognitive skills (e.g., short-term memory), and to show physical and mental endurance. As such, this apparatus may address some of the deficits targeted by conventional methods, but may do so with a wider, more active visual training environment, and by placing higher demands on integrated visuo-motor and visuo-cognitive functions (Klavora, 1995). A pilot study by Klavora et al. (1995), found that Dynavision training showed some rehabilitative promise for improving driving and basic psychomotor skills but recommended that future research on the benefits and limitations of Dynavision be explored. A follow-up study found that the performance score on several Dynavision tasks differentiated between persons who passed or failed an on-road driving assessment (Klavora, 2000). This study also compared the predictive validity of Dynavision and another off-road driving assessment device, the CBDI (Cognitive Behavioral Driver's Inventory; see description below). The researchers concluded that Dynavision would be of value in clinics that did not have driving programs or CBDI software. In those clinics, persons with stroke could be screened on Dynavision to determine whether they would be candidates for referral to a driver rehabilitation program (Klavora, 2000).

DRIVING AFTER STROKE: COGNITIVE AND PERCEPTUAL SKILLS

Stroke can produce a variety of cognitive difficulties that can affect an individuals' ability to return to driving. Some of these include: slowed information processing speed, visuo-spatial and perceptual deficits, visual inattention, concentration, and reasoning difficulties. As a result, cognition and driving after stroke has been extensively studied, with the main goals being to better define this relationship and to identify potential cognitive predictors of driving performance. To date, research has not been able to define a specific cognitive impairment pattern that is predictive of driving performance, but the results of these studies have identified specific cognitive domains relevant to driving and have also generated some new computerized and non-computerized driving assessment tasks, designed to better assess the cognitive domains of driving after stroke.

One of the most common problems associated with stroke and a cognitive domain identified from early on as relevant to driving is perceptual abilities (e.g., Sivak et al., 1981; Quigley & DeLisa, 1983). Early studies examining perceptual/cognitive abilities among right- and left-hemisphere stroke survivors indicated that individuals with right-hemisphere strokes demonstrated the most severe perceptual difficulties. Of those that returned to driving, when self-reported traffic difficulties (e.g., accident involvement) was examined 1 year later, the researchers reported the predictive validity of the perceptual assessment procedure held true for approximately 80% of the sample (Simms, 1985).

Another study, used a factor analysis approach to better define the perceptual–cognitive constructs of driving performance by conducting a comprehensive neuropsychological battery on 72 consecutively referred patients who had suffered a stroke (Sundet et al., 1995). The test battery was factor analyzed into 4 valid principal components; (1) visual perception, (2) spatial attention, (3) visuo-spatial processing, and (4) language/praxis. The researchers reported greater visual neglect in right-hemisphere strokes when compared to left-hemisphere strokes, but did not find overall group differences in the number of patients denied driving after the stroke. They concluded that, in addition to hemianopia, measures of neglect, speed of mental processing and emotional disturbances, such as denial-of-illness, showed to be the most potent subject characteristics in assessing patients for return to driving (Sundet et al., 1995).

One widely used neuropsychological assessment tool that attempts to capture perceptual–cognitive performance that is commonly used in driving assessment is the Motor-Free Visual Perceptual Task (MVPT). The MVPT is a standardized test of visual perception that was developed as an alternative to typical measures of visual perception which requires the subject to make graphemic responses (e.g., tracing or copying) and which, therefore, measures visuo-motor integration (MVPT-R Manual, 1995). As such, during the MVPT the examinee is instructed to look at a stimulus and then select the best option from four alternate figures to complete the item, without any motor involvement.

The MVPT is one of the most, if not the most (in some clinician's opinion), strongest predictor of on-road evaluation failure. In fact, in a survey of driving evaluation professionals conducted by Korner-Bitensky et al. (2006) found that the most commonly used perceptual–cognitive assessments in clinical settings were the MVPT (73%), followed by the Trail Making Test (TMT) (43%). The TMT can be best defined as a test of speed for attention, sequencing, mental flexibility, and of visual search and motor function (Spreen & Strauss, 1998). This task consists of two parts: Trails part A which is commonly viewed as a measure of simple attention and visual scanning and Trails part B, a more complex timed task, that requires the subject alternating between randomly arranged numbers and letters sequentially (1 – A – 2 – B – 3 – C, etc.). Even though Trails A and B are often administered together, Trails part B is more commonly utilized in driving assessment as it has been demonstrated to be indicative of driving performance in other clinical populations (e.g., dementia, traumatic brain injury).

In 1998, Mazer et al. examined the use of perceptual tests (including the MVPT and Trails B) to predict driving performance in individuals with stroke. Driving performance was quantified as pass or fail outcome of an on-road driving evaluation which was conducted by an occupational therapist and was based on observed driving behaviors. Their results found that the MVPT was the most predictive of on-road performance (positive predictive value = 86.1%; negative predictive values = 58.3%) and that the combination of the MVPT and Trails B represented the most predictive and parsimonious model for predicting on-road performance (Mazer et al., 1998).

Other researchers have reported that a neuropsychological assessment including tests measuring dynamic cognitive processing and complex speed can be useful in assessing driving skills after stroke. For example, Lundqvist et al. (2000) reported that the Complex Reaction time, the Stroop Color-Word Test, the Listening Span task, and a computerized administration of the K-test were most associated with driving skills, as defined in both on-road and simulated driving performance. Similarly, other researchers have found that even though the MVPT is believed to be a strong predictor of on-road evaluation failure, its predictive validity is not sufficiently high to warrant its use as the sole screening tool in identifying those who are unfit to undergo an on-road evaluation (Korner-Bitensky et al., 2000).

As the challenge of determining driving capacity following a stroke has been acknowledged, it is not uncommon to find that many settings rely on a team of clinician's who evaluate varying aspects of the individual's ability (e.g., medical, cognitive, etc.). One retrospective study, which attempted to better define the contributing factors to a team's decision of driving ability examined 104 individuals who had suffered a first stroke (Akinwuntan et al., 2002). The researchers administered both a comprehensive pre-driving assessment and an on-road test. The pre-driving assessment included specific measures of vision (monocular vision, binocular vision, stereoscopy, kinetic vision), and a neuropsychological assessment consisting of eight different tests: Rey Complex Figure Test, UFOV, divided attention, flexibility, visual scanning, incompatability, visual field, and neglect (Akinwuntan et al., 2002). Using logistic regression, the researchers found that a model including side of lesion, kinetic vision, visual scanning and a road test was the predictor of the team decision; and within that model the road test was the most important determinant. A combination of visual acuity and the Rey Complex Figure test was the best subset to predict on-road test performance (Akinwuntan et al., 2002). In follow-up prospective studies, these researchers found that a combination of visual neglect, Rey figure and on-road test was the best predictor of fitness to drive (as defined by clinician's ratings) (Akinwuntan et al., 2006). The accuracy of this short battery has recently been confirmed in another study demonstrating an 86% predictive value of these three tests, which are both sensitive (77%) and specific (92%) in their prediction (Akinwuntan et al., 2007).

Taken together, these studies clearly indicate that the determination of driving after stroke can not be limited to a single cognitive domain. Not surprising, these studies have led to the development of several composite tests that are designed to help clinicians assess the various cognitive domains relevant to driving. A brief description of three such batteries are provided below:

1. *Cognitive Behavioral Driver's Inventory* (Engum et al., 1988; Engum et al., 1989; Engum & Scott, 1990): The Cognitive Behavioral Driver's Inventory (CBDI) is a computerized neuropsychological test battery that has been designed to help rehabilitation professionals assess the cognitive and behavioral skills integral to the safe operation of a motor vehicle. The CBDI is standardized and includes norms and decision-making rules that have been developed in individuals with brain injury and normal controls. Although several studies have examined the validity of the CBDI, a recent study which focused on stroke found that the CBDI was predictive of driving outcome only in those individuals with

right-hemisphere strokes (Bouillon et al., 2006). The researchers also concluded that the CBDI was not sufficiently predictive of outcome to replace a driving evaluation.

2. *Sensory-Motor and Cognitive Tests* (Jones, 2006; Innes et al., 2007): The Sensory-Motor and Cognitive Tests (SMCTests) is a battery of computerized tests designed to quantify dysfunction in sensory-motor and cognitive performance, with a particular application to the assessment of driving available in patients with neurological disorder. The SMCTests is comprised of tests of visuo-perception, ballistic movement, and visuo-motor tracking; which have been extensively used as a standalone battery. A recent study by Innes et al. (2007) examined the ability of the SMCTests to predict driving performance (pass/fail performance on an on-road evaluation) in a group of 50 experienced drivers with brain disorders. Using binary logistic regression and non-linear causal resource analysis, the researchers reported that SMCTests had the highest predictive accuracy against "true on-road" driving ability (Innes et al., 2007).

3. *Stroke Driver Screening Assessment* (Nouri & Lincoln, 1992; Lincoln & Fanthome, 1994; Radford & Lincoln, 2004): The Stroke Driver Screening Assessment (SDSA) is a test battery which has been found to be predictive of stroke patients performance on road tests (Nouri & Lincoln, 1992). It consists of three tests: (1) Dot cancellation (visual inattention and concentration), (2) What's in the square? (reasoning ability), and (3) Road sign recognition. These three tests were identified from an earlier study which had included a broader test battery but had identified these three as the most predictive. Studies have examined both the reliability of the SDSA (Lincoln & Fanthome, 1994) and more recently, the concurrent validity of the SDSA. In the latter, tests of visuo-spatial ability which had been previously shown to be important determinants of driving, and not actual driving tasks or performance, were used as the driving criterion. Not surprisingly, correlations between these visuo-spatial tests and the SDSA were found, indicating that the SDSA appeared to measure predominantly attention and executive functions. To date, both a British and a Nordic version of the SDSA have been developed and continue to be evaluated (Lundberg et al., 2003).

In conclusion, the existing research on the cognitive demands of driving after stroke has consistently identified several domains as important predictors of driving capacity. Among these, visuo-spatial and/or perceptual–cognitive skills are of particular concerns for drivers after stroke, especially those with right-hemisphere stroke. Other areas, such as attention, information processing, and executive functions have also been examined and are consistent with findings in other clinical populations.

Yet, despite these findings, most of these studies are still limited by a common challenge in driving research, and that is the determinations of an appropriate driving criterion or driving outcome measure. As can be seen by this brief review, many of these studies have defined driving performance as pass or fail on an on-road driving evaluation. Yet, these evaluations are commonly flawed with their own limitations, including lack of validity, subjectivity, and lack of standardization. There is little to no evidence that performance on an on-road driving evaluation is predictive of actual "real world" driving. In fact, it can be argued that the artificial and limited driving experiences (must be limited due to safety issues) are not representative of events that everyday drivers encounter (Schultheis & Mourant, 2001) and does not allow the opportunity to test the limits of an individuals' capabilities.

DEFINING DRIVING PERFORMANCE: ON-ROAD AND SIMULATION

THE CLINICAL ON-ROAD DRIVING ASSESSMENT

Despite having numerous limitations, the on-road driving evaluation is one of the most commonly used assessment methods. A point underscored by the findings from Korner-Bitensky's survey of occupational therapy practices, which found that a client is usually put on the road for testing, regardless of how poorly he or she performed on the perceptual–cognitive tasks (Korner-Bitensky, 2006). The reasoning behind this practice was that clinicians felt that it was impossible to predict on the road performance, regardless of cognitive test performance, and that families would not accept the revocation of a driver's license without an on-road test.

However, it should be noted, that one group of Belgium researchers have focused extensively on the on-road driving evaluation and have demonstrated both reliability and validity of a standardized on-road driving evaluation. Specifically, these researchers identified a standard route and developed criteria for judging driver performance using a 13 item (49 subitems) checklist (Akinwuntan et al., 2003; Akinwuntan et al., 2005). Using these, evaluators make a determination of whether the individual is (a) fit to drive, (b) temporarily unfit to drive, or (c) definitively unfit to drive. A first study using three evaluators and video-recording was conducted to demonstrate the inter-rater reliability of this approach (Akinwuntan et al., 2003). A more recent study examined criterion validity, by comparing performance on this road test with performance on the Stroke Driver Screening Assessment (SDSA), where they reported agreement of performance between the two measures (Akinwuntan et al., 2005). While additional research is needed to further evaluate the relationship between the on-road and other measures of driving performance (e.g., actual traffic accidents or violations), this research clearly demonstrates that standardization of the on-road evaluation can greatly improve the value of the data collected. Unfortunately, while these researchers develop these methods for Belgium drivers, in the United States this task is more challenging given the fact that there is a lack of federal regulations regarding what defines an on-road evaluation. As such, most clinical sites conduct their own version of an on-road evaluation, which unfortunately leads to great variability in what it means to "pass" or "fail" an on-road test.

DRIVING SIMULATION ASSESSMENT

As an alternative and often in conjunction with on-road driving evaluations, the use of a driving simulator can offer several unique advantages to determining driving readiness. For example, driving simulations can allow clinicians to offer repeatable, standardized evaluations of driving performance in a variety of challenging driving scenarios that can be tailored to the individuals level of impairment (for complete discussion, see Chapter 11). In fact, in early studies of assessing driving after stroke, researchers reported the beneficial use of driving simulation as part of a comprehensive, multi-level driving evaluation (Quigley & DeLisa, 1983; Nouri & Tinson, 1988).

More recent work examining the use of driving simulation and stroke drivers has focused on the use of these systems to better identify specific differences in driving capacity in different types of strokes. For example, Kotterba et al., compared performance on neuropsychological tests (relevant to driving) and simulator driving in a group of individuals with acute ischemia in the middle cerebral artery (MCA) and in the vertebral artery (VA) and matched healthy controls. The findings indicated that although all patients had only mild deficits, the MCA ischemia patients demonstrated poorer results in the driving simulator and in accident rates (Kotterba et al., 2005). The researchers concluded that driving simulation assess various physical and neuropsychological functions that influence driving, even in mildly impaired populations and thus may tap into demands of driving not measured in more traditional driving assessment tools. A point that is shared by other researchers using driving simulation in other clinical populations (e.g., Schultheis et al., 2006).

DRIVING AND STROKE: OTHER INFLUENCING FACTORS

In addition to the discussed cognitive and physical impairments that may influence driving after a stroke, there are additional factors that require consideration and may further hinder an individual's ability to return to driving.

EMOTIONAL IMPAIRMENT AND SELF-AWARENESS

Individuals who are unable to drive may suffer increased isolation which may contribute to depression. Besides the physical limitations that can affect one's life after stroke, their professional and personal lives are also tested and stressed. Many people who have suffered from stroke are unable to return to work in the same capacity that they were prior to their disability. The disability not only affects the inflicted person, but also affects the person's close inner circle. For example, more dependence upon spouses/family members/close friends occurs for basic everyday activities such as eating, personal hygiene, and dressing.

It is also well-known that stroke patients may have problems in recognizing their own cognitive or psychomotor disorders, and may have serious impairment of functions which are crucial in safe driving. Particularly, damage to the non-dominant hemisphere often causes anosognosia and neglect syndrome and hence – lowered awareness. Heikkilä et al., found that the patients themselves and their spouses had a clear tendency to overestimate driving ability (when compared to the estimates of the neurologist and psychologist) (Heikkilä et al., 1999).

AGING AND STROKE

In addition to coping with residual deficits of a stroke, many older adults must cope with ongoing cognitive and physical changes that are commonly seen in aging adults. For example, decreased physical mobility, changes in vision, changes in cognition (e.g., memory problems). Older individuals are also at risk for other neurological involvement, they may be at risk for additional strokes, other cardiovascular disorders and/or heightened risk for injuries.

EDUCATION (FOR THE PATIENT AND FOR THE CLINICIAN)

In even the earliest study conducted by Quigley (1983), part of the rehabilitation team's efforts is directed toward providing the candidate with information about Department of Motor Vehicle (DMV) policies and restrictions. But, in a study by Kelly et al. (1999), investigating the awareness of patients and doctors of medical restrictions to driving, the researchers found that educating the client may be difficult. Besides patients having difficulty knowing if they should drive based on their medical condition, Kelly et al., found that doctors' knowledge of the current licensing policy and action to be taken if a patient was not eligible to drive was very poor. Medical staff do not seem to be able to provide this guidance. To increase the awareness of doctors of medical restrictions to driving, greater emphasis must be placed on this aspect of patient care during both undergraduate and postgraduate training (Kelly et al., 1999).

In conclusion, the current chapter attempts to provide a review of the literature that has studied driving after a stroke. From this, the following points can be made:

- Currently there are no universally accepted guidelines for what constitutes a complete assessment of an individual for determining the ability to return to driving.
- Off-road tests of vision and visual attention, including visual scanning and visual information processing, can serve to determine an individuals' readiness for on-road assessment.
- Off-road tests of attention, information processing, working memory, spatio-perception, and visuo-perceptual skills can serve to determine an individuals' readiness for on-road assessment.

- Evidence does not support the use of one assessment for determining the ability to drive safely, multiple assessments are recommended (e.g., off-road, on-road, driving simulation).
- Side of lesion does not significantly predict driving outcome, but there is evidence supporting greater difficulties in individuals with right-hemisphere involvement.
- There are several comprehensive driver assessment batteries that can aid in predicting on-road driving fitness with reasonable accuracy.
- Evidence supports future use of off-road driving simulators for assessment of ability to return to driving post-CVA. Simulators have the potential to be an economical and efficient clinical tool.
- The most commonly used driving outcome measures is the on-road driving assessment which is fraught with numerous limitations, including overdependence on subjective observations, lack of standardization and does not allow challenging assessment to establish the individuals capacity limits.
- Future research is needed to better define accurate driving criterion or driving outcome measures. Current criterion may or may not be representative of "real world" driving performance.
- Additional factors, such as limited self-awareness, emotional stability, and aging must also be considered in determining the individual's capacity to continue driving.

REFERENCES

Akinwuntan, A. E., Feys, H., DeWeerdt, W., Pauwels, J., Baten, G., & Strypstein, E. (2002). Determinants of driving after stroke. *Arch. Phys. Med. Rehabil.*, *3*(3), 334–341.

Akinwuntan, A. E., DeWeerdt, W., Feys, H., Baten, G., Arno, P., & Kiekens, C. (2003). Reliability of a road test after stroke. *Arch. Phys. Med. Rehabil.*, *84*(12), 1792–1796.

Akinwuntan, A. E., De Weerdt, W., Feys, H., Pauwels, J., Baten, G., Arno, P., & Kiekens, C. (2005). Effect of simulator training on driving after stroke: A randomized controlled trial. *Neurology*, *65*(6), 843–850.

Akinwuntan, A. E., De Weerdt, W., Feys, H., Baten, G., Arno, P., & Kiekens, C. (2005). The validity of a road test after stroke. *Arch. Phys. Med. Rehabil.*, *86*(3), 421–426.

Akinwuntan, A. E., Feys, H., De Weerdt, W., Baten, G., Arno, P., & Kiekens, C. (2006). Prediction of driving after stroke: A prospective study. *Neurorehabil. Neural Repair*, *20*(3), 417–423.

Akinwuntan, A. E., Devos, H., Feys, H., Verheyden, G., Baten, G., Kiekens, C., & De Weerdt, W. (2007). Confirmation of the accuracy of a short battery to predict fitness-to-drive of stroke survivors without severe deficits. *J. Rehabil. Med.*, *39*(9), 698–702.

Ball, K., Owsley, C., Sloane, M. E., Roenker, D. L., & Bruni, J. R. (1993). Visual attention problems as a predictor of vehicle crashes in older drivers. *Invest. Ophthalmol. Vis. Sci.*, *34*(11), 3110–3123.

Bouillon, L., Mazer, B., & Gelinas, I. (2006). Validity of the cognitive behavioral driver's inventory in predicting out-come. *Am. J. Occup. Ther.*, *60*, 420–427.

Carter, T., & Major, H. (2003). Driving restrictions after stroke: Doctors' awareness of DVLA guidelines and advice given to patients. *Clin. Med.*, *3*(2), 187.

Engum, E. S., & Lambert, E. W. (1990). Restandardization of the cognitive behavioral driver's inventory. *Cognit. Rehabil.*, *8*, 20–27.

Engum, E. S., Womac, J., Pendergrass, T., & Lambert, E. W. (1988). Norms and decision making rules for the cognitive behavioral driver's inventory. *Cognit. Rehabil.*, *6*, 12–16.

Engum, E. S., Pendergrass, T. M., Cron, L., Lambert, E. W., & Hulse, C. K. (1988). Cognitive behavioral driver's inventory. *Cognit. Rehabil.*, *6*, 34–48.

Engum, E. S., Pendergrass, T. M., Cron, L., Lambert, W., & Hulse, C. K. (1989). Criterion-related validity of the cognitive behavioral driver's index. *Cognit. Rehabil.*, *7*, 22–30.

Fisk, G. D., & Mennemeier, M. (2006). Common neuropsychological deficits associated with stroke survivors' impaired performance on a useful field of view test. *Percept. Mot. Skills.*, *102*(2), 387–394.

Fisk, G. D., Owlsey, C., & Pulley, L. V. (1997). Driving after stroke: Driving exposure, advice, and evaluations. *Arch. Phys. Med. Rehabil.*, *78*(12), 1338–1345.

Fisk, G. D., Owsley, C., & Mennemeier, M. (2002). Vision, attention, and self-reported driving behaviors in community-dwelling stroke survivors. *Arch. Phys. Med. Rehabil.*, *83*(4), 469–477.

Gilhotra, J. S., Mitchell, P., Healey, P. R., Cumming, R. G., & Currie, J. (2002). Homonymous visual field defects and stroke in an older population. *Stroke, 33*, 2417–2420.

Heikkilä, V. M., Korpelainen, J., Turkka, J., Kallanranta, T., & Summala, H. (1999). Clinical evaluation of the driving ability in stroke patients. *Acta Neurol. Scand.*, *6*, 349–355.

Innes, C. R., Jones, R. D., Dalrymple-Alford, J. C., Hayes, S., Hollobon, S., Severinsen, J., Smith, G., Nicholls, A., & Anderson, T. J. (2007). Sensory-motor and cognitive tests predict driving ability of persons with brain disorders. *J. Neurol.*, *260*(1–2), 188–198.

Jones, R. (2006). *Measurement of Sensory-Motor Control Performance Capacities: Tracking Tasks.* Boca Raton, Florida: CRC Press.

Kelly, R., Warke, T., & Steele, I. (1999). Medical restrictions to driving: the awareness of patients and doctors. *Postgrad. Med. J.*, *75*(887), 537–539.

Khan, S., De Silva, D., & Mohanaruban, K. (2003). Driving restrictions after stroke: doctors' awareness of DVLA guidelines and advice given to patients. *Clin. Med.*, *3*(2), 187.

Klavora, P., Gaskovski, P., Martin, K., Forsyth, R. D., Heslegrave, R. J., Young, M., & Quinn, R. (1995). The effects of dynavision rehabilitation on behind-the-wheel driving ability and selected psychomotor abilities of persons after stroke. *Am. J. Occup. Ther.*, *49*(6), 534–542.

Klavora, P., Heslegrave, R. J., & Young, M. (2000). Driving skills in elderly persons with stroke: Comparison of two new assessment options. *Arch. Phys. Med. Rehabil.*, *81*(6), 701–705.

Korner-Bitensky, N., Mazer, B., Sofer, S. et al. (2000). Visual testing for readiness to drive: A multi-center study. *Am. J. Phy. Med. Rehabil.*, *79*, 253–259.

Korner-Bitensky, N., Bitensky, J., Sofer, S., Man-Son-Hing, M., & Gelinas, I. (2006). Driving evaluation practices of clinicians working in the United States and Canada. *Am. J. Occup. Ther.*, *60*(4), 428–434.

Kotterba, S., Widdig, W., Brylak, S., & Orth, M. (2005). Driving after cerebral ischemia – A driving simulator investigation. *Wien Med Wochenschr.*, *155*(15–16), 348–353.

Lee, N., Tracy, J., Bohannon, R. W., & Ahlquist, M. (2003). Driving resumption and its predictors after stroke. *Conn. Med.*, *67*(7), 387–391.

Legh-Smith, J., Wade, D. T., & Langton, H. R. (1986). Driving after stroke. *J. R. Soc. Med.*, *79*, 200–2003.

Lincoln, N. B., & Fanthome, Y. (1994). Reliability of the stroke drivers screening assessment. *Clin. Rehabil.*, *8*, 157–160.

Lister, R. (1999). Loss of ability to drive following a stroke: The early experiences of three elderly people on discharge from hospital. *Stroke*, *62*(11), 1499–1505.

Lundberg, C., Caneman, G., Samuelsson, S. M., Hakamies-Blomqvist, L., & Almkvist, O. (2003). The assessment of fitness to drive after a stroke: The Nordic Stroke Driver Screening Assessment. *Scand. J. Psychol.*, *44*(1), 23–30.

Lundqvist, A., Gerdle, B., & Ronnberg, J. (2000). Neuropsychological aspects of driving after stroke – in the simulator and on the road. *Appl. Cognit. Psychol.*, *14*, 135–150.

Marshall, S. C., Molnar, F., Man-Son-Hing, M., Blair, R., Brosseau, L., Finestone, H. M., Lamothe, C., Korner-Bitensky, N., & Wilson, K. G. (2007). Predictors of driving ability following stroke: A systematic review. *Top Stroke Rehabil.*, *14*(1), 98–114.

Mazer, BL., Korner-Bitensky, N., & Sofer, S. (1998). Predicting ability to drive after stroke. *Arch. Phys. Med. Rehabil.*, *79*(7), 743–750.

Mazer, B. L., Sofer, S., Korner-Bitensky, N., & Gelinas, I. (2001). Use of the UFOV to evaluate and retrain visual attention skills in clients with stroke: A pilot study. *Am. J. Occup. Ther.*, *55*(5), 552–557.

Mazer, B. L., Sofer, S., Korner-Bitensky, N., Gelinas, I., Hanley, J., & Wood-Dauphinee, S. (2003). Effectiveness of a visual attention retraining program on the driving performance of clients with stroke. *Arch. Phys. Med. Rehabil.*, *84*(4), 541–550.

Millar, W. J. (1999). Older drivers– A complex public health issue. *Health Rep.*, *11*(2), 59–71.

Nouri, F. M., & Lincoln, N. B. (1992). Validation of a cognitive assessment: Predicting driving performance after stroke. *Clin. Rehabil.*, *6*, 275–281.

Nouri, F. M., & Tinson, D. J. (1988). A comparison of a driving simulator and a road test in the assessment of driving ability after a stroke. *Clin. Rehabil.*, *2*, 99–104.

Quigley, F. L., & DeLisa, J. L. (1983). Assessing the driving potential of cerebral vascular accident patients. *Am. J. Occup. Ther.*, *37*(7), 474–478.

Radford, K. A., & Lincoln, N. B. (2004). Concurrent validity of the stroke drivers screening assessment. *Arch. Phys. Med. Rehabil.*, *85*(2), 324–328.

Radford, K. A., Lincoln, N. B., & Murray-Leslie, C. (2004). Validation of the stroke drivers screening assessment for people with traumatic brain injury. *Brain Inj.*, *18*(8), 775–786.

Roaf, E., & Jankowiak, J. (2005). Patient page. Driving after a stroke: What helps grandma drive safely? *Neurology*, *65*(6), E13–E14.

Samuelsson, S. M. (2005). Physicians' control of driving after stroke attacks. *Tidsskr Nor Laegeforen*, *125*(19), 2610–2612.

Schultheis, M. T., & Mourant, R. R. (2001). Virtual reality and driving: The road to better assessment of cognitively impaired populations. *Presence: Teleoperators and Virtual Environments*, *10*(4), 436–444.

Schultheis, M. T., Simone, L. K., Roseman, E., Nead, R., Rebimbas, J., & Mourant, R. (2006). Stopping behavior in a VR driving simulator: A new clinical measure for the assessment of driving? *IEEE Eng. Med. Biol. Sci.*, 4921–4924.

Simms, B. (1985). Perception and driving: Theory and practice. *Br. J. Occup. Ther.*, *48*, 363–366.

Sivak, O., Kewman, W., & Henson, (1981). Driving and perceptual/cognitive skills; Behavioral consequences of brain damage. *Arch. Phys. Med. Rehabil.*, *62*, 476–483.

Smith-Arena, L., Edelstein, L., & Rabadi, M. H. (2006). Predictors of a successful driver evaluation in stroke patients after discharge based on an acute rehabilitation hospital evaluation. *Am. J. Phys. Med. Rehabil.*, *85*(1), 44–52.

Söderström, S. T., Pettersson, R. P., & Leppert, J. (2006). Prediction of driving ability after stroke and the effect of behind-the-wheel training. *Scand. J. Psychol.*, *47*(5), 4129.

Spreen, O., & Strauss, E. (1991). *A Compendium of Neuropsychological Tests: Administration, Norms, and Commentary*. NY: Oxford University Press.

Sundet, K., Goffeng, L., & Hofft, E. (1995). To drive or not to drive: Neuropsychological assessment for driver's license among stroke patients. *Scand. J. Psychol.*, *36*, 47–58.

8

DRIVING AND OTHER NEUROLOGICAL AND PSYCHIATRIC DISORDERS

JESSICA H. KALMAR AND JOHN DeLUCA

The privilege of driving an automobile has become an essential ingredient for communal integration in today's society. The vast majority of individuals rely upon vehicular transportation for social and occupational functions, as well as other activities of daily living. However, this privilege is contingent upon competence in certain areas, such as visual, physical and cognitive abilities. For instance, cognitive impairment due to brain dysfunction can significantly affect one's ability to operate a motor vehicle and may result in the loss of this privilege. Relationships between such cognitive dysfunction and driving impediments have been demonstrated in individuals with traumatic brain injury, people with dementing conditions, and those who have suffered from cerebral vascular accidents. The impact of these conditions on driving is addressed in other chapters in this volume.

The present chapter addresses the impact of attention-deficit/hyperactivity disorder (ADHD), multiple sclerosis (MS), epilepsy and psychiatric disorders on individuals' driving capacity. While the research on driving and both ADHD and MS is limited, epilepsy and psychiatric conditions have been investigated more extensively within the driving literature. For each disorder, a brief description of the illness and its associated cognitive and physical difficulties will be provided, followed by a discussion of how the condition might impact the ability to operate a motor vehicle. The existing literature on driving and the specific disorder will be reviewed and critiqued. Issues covered in the existing literature include rates of negative driving behaviors, risks for poor driving outcomes, and legal issues pertinent to automobile driving for each disease population. Finally, suggestions for future research are provided.

ATTENTION-DEFICIT/HYPERACTIVITY DISORDER

ADHD is a childhood psychiatric diagnosis characterized by symptomatology across three behavioral domains: inattention, overactivity, and impulsivity (American Psychiatric Association, 1994). Behaviors in the realm of inattention include: difficulty maintaining attention over time, difficulty completing tasks, being forgetful, easily distracted and disorganized, not listening, making careless mistakes, avoiding tasks that require concentration, and frequently losing things. Symptoms of overactivity and impulsivity include being fidgety, noisy and "constantly on the go," interrupting others, running around excessively, and having difficulty staying seated or waiting in line. In order to meet criteria for diagnosis of the disorder, symptoms must begin before the age of seven, be present substantially more often than in children of the same age and gender, cause impairment in functioning and be present across settings (i.e., not confined to only school or only home). Prevalence of the disorder in childhood is estimated at 3–5% (American Psychiatric Association, 1994). Traditionally, cognitive impairment in ADHD was thought to be associated with an inability to attend during social and academic tasks (Douglas, 1983). However, more recently, investigators have suggested that the cognitive correlates of ADHD are principally accounted for by deficits in executive function (Barkley, 1997).

A body of evidence has accumulated suggesting that ADHD persists into adulthood in 30–60% of childhood-onset cases (Marks et al., 2001). Behaviors found in adults with ADHD, which may impact upon one's ability to operate a motor vehicle, include inattention, behavioral disinhibition, motor dyscontrol, and executive dysfunction. Furthermore, substance abuse, antisocial behavior, and excessive risk taking are amongst the risk factors that have been proposed for motor vehicle collisions (MVCs) (Lapham et al., 2001) and are more likely to be exhibited by adults with ADHD than healthy controls (Hechtman & Weiss, 1986). Thus, adolescents and adults with ADHD could be prone to a higher frequency of MVCs than the general population. The high incidence of death related to MVC amongst adolescents (US Department of Education, 1988), combined with the potentially increased risk for impaired driving amongst individuals with ADHD, have recently led to investigations of the driving habits of adolescents and adults with ADHD.

A longitudinal study conducted by Barkley et al. (1993) followed children with ADHD and healthy controls into early adulthood and compared their driving-related behaviors in order to explore driving risks associated with ADHD. Average age for the ADHD participants was 19.1 years. Driving outcome measures obtained in this study were limited to parental report collected via survey and rating scales. According to parental report, individuals with ADHD had more negative driving outcomes than healthy controls in all areas that were questioned. These included safe driving habits, MVCs, physical injuries sustained during MVCs, demonstrating fault for an MVC, traffic citations, driving an automobile illegally, and suspension or cancellation of driving licenses. Barkley et al. (1993) attempted to determine the specific component of ADHD that contributed to poor driving outcomes. Data indicated that ADHD participants who presented with comorbid symptoms of oppositional defiant disorder (ODD) and conduct disorder (CD) at follow-up exhibited the greatest risk for negative driving outcomes. However, due to the similarity of symptoms in individuals with ADHD, ODD and CD, it was not possible to isolate the independent contributions of these disorders to negative driving outcomes in this sample.

A second study of the relationship between ADHD and driving behaviors conducted by Barkley's group (Murphy & Barkley, 1996) extended their original efforts by sampling a population of adults with ADHD (mean age = 32 years) and comparing their driving behaviors to that of a mixed clinical and healthy control group. The control group was comprised of adults with mood and anxiety disorders (50%), self-referred adults who did not receive any diagnoses (40%) and a mixture of individuals diagnosed with substance dependence or dementia not otherwise specified. Information on driving behaviors was obtained via interview of the participant. According to self-report of driving behavior, adults with ADHD exhibited greater driving risk, in the form of more speeding violations, and had a higher number of driving license suspensions and MVCs than the clinical/healthy control group. These data indicate that driving risk associated with ADHD is not limited to adolescence or early adulthood, rather it extends into later adulthood. Furthermore, driving risk was reported to be specific to ADHD, rather than a general correlate of psychiatric illness as the individuals with ADHD exhibited more driving risk than the clinical/healthy control group (Murphy & Barkley, 1996). Limitations of this study include the heterogeneous nature of the control group as well as the subjective nature of the dependent variables (i.e., that information on driving was limited to that obtained via self-report measures).

Barkley et al.'s (Barkley et al., 1993; Murphy & Barkley, 1996) first investigations of driving behaviors in ADHD employed a rather narrow scope of dependent measures, that is, reports of driving history provided by participants and significant others. In an effort to collect more in-depth information on, and examine more quantitative factors of, driving behaviors, Barkley et al. (1996) compared the official driving records of young adults with ADHD and healthy controls. The young adults (between 17 and 30 years of age) with and without ADHD also completed a written test of driving knowledge following video presentations and a test of driving skills in the form of a driving simulator. Finally, reports of driving history were obtained from the participants and their significant others. The two subject groups did not differ in extent of prior driving experience, a confounding factor that had not been addressed in the earlier studies (Barkley et al., 1993; Murphy & Barkley, 1996). Consistent with earlier data (Barkley et al., 1993; Murphy & Barkley, 1996), ADHD participants had more speeding citations and license suspensions, were involved in more MVCs, were more likely to have experienced MVCs that caused bodily injury, and were reported to have fewer safe driving habits relative to healthy controls. Regarding the driving simulation used to measure skill, ADHD subjects displayed more crashes, scrapes, and erratic steering than healthy controls. There were no group differences on the written test of driving knowledge. These data suggest that driving difficulties in ADHD are related to impaired driving skills rather than insufficient driving knowledge.

In summary, the work of Barkley's group consistently shows that individuals with ADHD are at greater risk for unlawful and unsafe driving behaviors, resulting in more traffic citations, MVCs, and license suspensions, than healthy controls. The work by this group suggests that interventions for the ADHD population should be geared toward improving driving practices and should be shaped by research demonstrating impaired driving skills rather than deficient driving knowledge.

Additional support for ADHD in childhood functioning as a risk factor for poor automobile driving in early adulthood (through 25 years of age) is cited in the Notes of the National Highway Traffic Safety Administration (NHTSA, 1997). A longitudinal study described by the NHTSA found that individuals who present with severe ADHD in childhood, as compared to those with mild ADHD symptomatology and healthy controls, were more likely to be convicted of assorted moving and non-moving traffic violations from the time they received their driving license through age 25. However, the two groups did not differ in incidence of MVCs from the time they received their driving licenses through 25 years of age. While the similar rate of MVCs across subject groups diverges from the earlier findings of Barkley's group, it is noteworthy that the longitudinal study reported by the NHTSA utilized a control group that contained a mixture of healthy controls and individuals with mild ADHD symptomatology. The NHTSA theorize that poor impulse control may be the underlying factor in the driving difficulties evidenced in ADHD and describes several intervention strategies, including administration of stimulant medication, early identification of at-risk populations, and implementation of a graduated licensing program. However, no data were presented to support the idea that impaired impulse control is responsible for driving difficulties in ADHD.

Given the evidence for the association between ADHD and negative driving behaviors, Cox et al. (2000) investigated the efficacy of methylphenidate, a stimulant medication commonly used for the treatment of ADHD, for potentially enhancing driving performance in individuals with ADHD. A double-blind placebo controlled crossover design was conducted comparing the performance of young adults with and without ADHD on a driving simulator test pre- and post-administration of methylphenidate or placebo. An index of impairment on the driving simulator test was compiled using information recorded on steering, braking, and crashes. Consistent with prior research, ADHD participants reported more MVCs and traffic citations than control subjects and exhibited impaired performance on the driving simulator test in the baseline condition relative to healthy controls. Administration of a single dose of methylphenidate engendered significant improvement in driving simulator performance of the ADHD subjects, such that their scores reached the level of healthy control performance. No change was seen in driving simulator performance of healthy controls following administration of methylphenidate.

Most recently, Barkley's group (2002) attempted to further delineate the specific aspects of ADHD that contribute to negative driving behavior and included assessment of the cognitive correlates of driving behavior. Michon's (1985) multifactorial model of driving was utilized in selecting the basic cognitive components of driving behavior to be evaluated. Comprehensive assessment of driving behavior included self-report, parental report, official records from the Department of Motor Vehicles, cognitive testing, driving simulator test, and a test of driving knowledge. Consistent with prior research, young adults with ADHD (ages 17–28) had more traffic citations, experienced more MVCs, and had more frequent license suspensions than community controls. However, in contrast to earlier work, individuals with ADHD exhibited weaker driving knowledge and intact driving simulator performance, relative to the control group. The authors suggested that these discrepant findings were reflective of the measures chosen and did not represent an actual departure from earlier reported findings. Regarding the driving simulator, the authors theorized that the simple simulator used in this study was inadequate to detect the subtle difficulties that young adults with ADHD may have when operating a motor vehicle.

Results of correlational analysis indicated a limited relationship between cognition and driving. That is, performance on measures of executive functions was modestly related to MVC frequency and total traffic violations. Driving difficulties were not shown to be a function of comorbid conditions, including ODD, depression, anxiety or frequent alcohol/drug use. When interviewed about factors that may have contributed to their MVCs, both subject groups reported that they believed inattention to be the most common contributor to their first and second automobile accidents. However, information gathered from objective cognitive testing in Barkley's study did not support this self-report.

Generally, ADHD research has predominantly male samples, as the disorder is much more frequent in males than females. Thus, the literature on driving behaviors in ADHD cited to this point has not been able to determine whether driving risks associated with ADHD vary across gender. Nada-Raja et al. (1997) conducted a longitudinal study of a birth cohort from New Zealand, which included a larger number of females than studies previously reported herein, and examined the driving patterns of females with ADHD. At age 15, the cohort was divided into four subject groups: those diagnosed with ADHD, those diagnosed with ODD or CD, those diagnosed with a mood or anxiety disorder, and a healthy control group. Results showed that degree of psychiatric symptomatology present at age 15 was associated with driving behavior at age 18, such that ADHD and CD symptoms at age 15 were both positively associated with driving offenses at age 18. However, amongst males, data indicated that relative to CD symptoms, ADHD symptoms made minimal contribution to prediction of driving offenses in this adolescent community sample. Conversely, amongst females, individuals with ADHD exhibited the worst driving outcomes, relative to the three female comparison groups. Thus, these data suggest different risk factors for negative driving outcomes across gender. ADHD symptomatology has a larger contribution to negative driving outcome than conduct problems in females, whereas amongst males CD symptoms are the strongest predictors of breaking driving regulations in adolescence.

Importantly, the study of Nada-Raja et al. (1997) showed that driving difficulties could not be entirely explained by ADHD symptomatology per se (i.e., inattention, overactivity, impulsivity). Rather, gender and the presence of conduct problems were shown to act as confounding factors. Additional potential confounds posited in the driving literature amongst individuals with ADHD and other illnesses include extent of prior driving experience, intelligence level, family functioning, and social background. A longitudinal study of a New Zealand community sample revealed a linear relationship between degree of attentional difficulties at age 13 and negative driving outcomes displayed between the ages of 18–21 (e.g., MVCs, drunk driving, and traffic violations) (Woodward et al., 2000). In this study, baseline psychiatric assessment was conducted via parent and teacher report, while driving outcome was measured through self-report on structured interview and rating scales. Gender, prior driving experience, and degree of conduct problems at age 13 were shown to be significant covariates, such that the association between early attentional difficulties and later driving outcomes was minimized when these factors were added to the analyses. After controlling for these confounding factors, the associations between attentional difficulties and some of the driving outcomes (e.g., non-injurious MVCs) were no longer significant. However, early attentional difficulties maintained a significant association with MVCs that resulted in injury as well as certain traffic violations. These results suggest that the individual at risk for the highest number of poor driving behaviors is the young male with CD who despite his limited driving experience drives often (Woodward et al., 2000).

In summary, all of the studies reviewed herein indicate an increased risk for some form of driving difficulty in individuals with ADHD relative to healthy controls. As depicted in Table 8.1, the range of observed driving difficulties included driving violations, license suspensions, and MVCs (see Table 8.1). Discrepant findings in the literature regarding some of the negative driving behaviors may be related to the methodological differences across studies or the heterogeneous nature of individuals with ADHD, particularly with regard to comorbid psychiatric difficulties. The majority of the studies, which investigated comorbid psychiatric disorders, reported that the negative driving behaviors

TABLE 8.1   Driving Behaviors Across Individuals with ADHD, MS, and Control Groups.

Study	Unsafe driving habits	MVC	MVC causing injury	Driving offenses	License suspension	Driving simulator	Driving knowledge
ADHD							
Barkley et al. (1993)	ADHD > HC	ADHD > HC	ADHD > HC	ADHD > HC	ADHD > HC	–	–
Murphy and Barkley (1996)	–	ADHD > MC	–	ADHD > MC	ADHD > MC	–	–
Barkley et al. (1996)	ADHD > HC	ADHD > HC	ADHD > HC	ADHD > HC	ADHD > HC	ADHD < HC	NS
NHTSA (1997)	–	NS	–	ADHD > MC	–	–	–
Cox et al. (2000)	–	ADHD > HC	–	ADHD > HC	–	ADHD < HC	–
Barkley et al. (2002)	–	ADHD > HC	–	ADHD > HC	ADHD > HC	NS	ADHD < HC
MS							
Knecht (1977)	–	MS > HC	–	MS > HC	–	–	–
Schultheis et al. (2002)	–	MSCI > HC	–	NS	–	–	–

– = Not assessed; HC = Healthy controls; MC = Mixed control group; NS = No significant differences; MSCI = MS cognitively impaired; ADHD = Attention-deficit/hyperactivity disorder; MS = Multiple sclerosis; MVC = Motor vehicle collision.

exhibited by individuals with ADHD were related to comorbidity in the realm of externalizing behaviors (e.g., ODD and CD) but not in the domain of internalizing behaviors (mood and anxiety disorders). Other factors, including gender, cognitive performance, and medication status, were also shown to play a role in the driving behaviors of individuals with ADHD. While driving research in the ADHD population is a relatively new endeavor, scientific advances with time are evident across the limited number of studies, including use of more objective dependent measures, larger sample sizes, and investigation of confounding factors. Limitations of the literature, which should be addressed in future research, include a short time window for assessment of driving behavior, difficulty comparing findings across studies due to differences in methodology, the lack of clarity regarding which component of ADHD contributes to poor driving behavior and poor integration with the literature on driving in other psychiatric conditions.

MULTIPLE SCLEROSIS

Multiple sclerosis (MS) is an inflammatory disease of the central nervous system, characterized by demyelinated plaques with a chronic and highly variable disease course. It is characterized by a waxing and waning progression due to destruction of the myelin sheath encasing neuronal axons throughout the central nervous system (Rao, 1986). Although demyelnation is the hallmark of the illness, more recently, evidence has accumulated demonstrating axonal damage as well (Trapp et al., 1998; Bitsch et al., 2000). Common symptoms of MS include motor impairment, sensory changes, cognitive problems, muscle weakness, and fatigue (Miller, 2001). MS can be experienced in mild forms or, alternatively, it may be expressed in a severe, progressive and debilitating fashion (Minden & Schiffer, 1990). The disease is more common in women than men and while the primary cause is unknown, both environmental and genetic factors have been postulated to be contributory (Pryse-Phillips & Costello, 2001).

Unlike several other neurologic conditions, few studies have examined driving skills and abilities in persons with MS. While physical impairment is viewed as a characteristic of MS that would impact upon driving ability, the influence of cognitive factors on driving ability has received little attention. Physical difficulties seen in individuals with MS that may affect driving behavior include limb weakness, spasticity, ataxia, incoordination, tremor, and visual impediments (Goodwill, 1984). It is only recently, given the emerging reports of cognitive dysfunction in MS in domains that have been shown to be central to driving capacity, that studies have begun to examine cognitive factors in driving ability in persons with MS. These cognitive factors include attention, visual perceptual skills, processing speed, and executive functions (DeLuca et al., 1994; DeLuca et al., 1998).

Knecht (1977) conducted the earliest investigation of driving behavior in individuals with MS. Given the course and clinical characteristics of MS, Knecht

(1977) theorized that individuals with MS would be poor drivers, relative to healthy controls. Following comparison of official records of traffic offenses and collisions of individuals with MS and healthy controls, Knecht (1977) reported that individuals with MS caused more MVCs and committed more driving offenses than healthy controls. It was recommended that a physician follow individuals with MS who hold valid driver's licenses regularly.

Although this initial report was compelling, the relationship between MS and driving received little further attention until 1995 when Schanke et al. examined the prerequisites for driving amongst 33 Norwegian patients with MS. A sample of individuals with MS underwent neuropsychological and medical testing, and a portion of the sample also completed a behind-the-wheel driving evaluation. Based on test results, a determination was made as to whether the individuals were fit to drive or not. Regression analyses revealed that cognitive and emotional dysfunction contributed more to driving fitness than illness duration and degree of neurological deficit. The authors suggested indicators for when assessment of driving skills is warranted and provided some guidelines for the assessment of prerequisites for a driver's license in Norway among individuals with MS.

The first attempt to directly study the impact of cognitive impairment on driving skills in persons with MS was conducted by Schultheis et al. (2001). Three subject groups were recruited: healthy controls, individuals with MS who exhibited cognitive impairment, and individuals with MS who were cognitively intact. All subjects with MS had a current valid driver's license and minimal physical disability. Inclusion was restricted to only MS subjects with minimal physical disability so that physical complications would not confound studying the effects of cognitive impairment on driving performance. The three groups were evaluated using two computerized measures of skills required for driving. The Useful Field of Vision (UFOV) test is a commercially available product that quantifies the visual field over which a driver can process rapidly presented visual information. The UFOV yields a score that suggests a level of driving risk for the participant. The Neurocognitive Driving Test (NDT) is a computer-based simulation based on real-world driving scenarios. The NDT assesses driving-related skills, including reaction time, visual spatial skills, driving knowledge, and performance on driving simulation, in an ecologically valid format (Schultheis et al., 2003). The results of this study showed that the group of MS participants with cognitive impairment performed significantly worse than the MS group without cognitive problems and healthy controls on two of the three portions of the UFOV and the latency to perform driving-specific functions on the NDT. This was the first systematic study to show that cognitive difficulties in persons with MS could affect driving performance.

In a second study conducted by Schultheis et al. (2002) examination of DMV records for this sample indicated that individuals with MS who were cognitively impaired had a higher incidence of MVCs when compared to healthy controls and individuals with MS who were cognitively intact. There were no group differences in motor vehicle violations. These data suggest the difference in MVC incidence across groups was not related to differential compliance with driving regulations. It is noteworthy that the cognitively impaired individuals with MS reported the lowest driving frequency across groups, and yet they still exhibited the highest rate of MVCs. This extension of their prior work used actual DMV record data to support the earlier finding that impaired cognitive functioning affects driving behaviors in the MS population.

In summary, despite the limited number of studies investigating driving behaviors in individuals with MS, data obtained from official records of motor vehicle departments and computerized measures across studies suggest that driving is impaired in at least some subset of individuals with MS (see Table 8.1). Furthermore, while cognitive dysfunction has been implicated with regard to these driving impairments, additional studies confirming and extending these initial investigations are clearly required. Larger sample sizes, confounding factors including level of disease expression, contribution of gender, specific cognitive factors, and differentiation between the effects of physical and cognitive impairments on driving in the MS population are areas to be addressed in future investigations.

EPILEPSY

Epilepsy is a neurological illness that is characterized by the occurrence of two or more electrophysiological seizures (Neppe & Tucker, 1988). Behavioral changes that accompany the seizure may include abnormal sensations, visual, olfactory or auditory hallucinations, fears, depression, staring spells, or convulsive movements, with the episodes lasting from seconds to minutes. Disturbances in consciousness, behavior and/or mood may occur before or after the seizures, or during the time period between seizures. The current epilepsy classification system differentiates between generalized epilepsies/syndromes and localization-related epilepsies/syndromes (Commission on Classification and Terminology of the International League Against Epilepsy, 1989). Generalized seizures begin in both hemispheres of the brain simultaneously (Devinsky, 1994). Localization-related epilepsies, on the other hand, are characterized by seizures that begin in a restricted brain region, though they often spread to other brain regions. Termed partial seizures, these tend to result in discrete symptoms that are quite similar with each recurring seizure, due to their origin in a restricted brain region. Partial seizures can further be divided into simple partial seizures and complex partial seizures. Awareness remains unaltered throughout simple partial seizures, whereas complex partial seizures are characterized by an alteration in awareness. Cognizance of the simple partial seizure by the individual is termed an aura. A wide variety of localization-related epilepsies exist, including temporal lobe epilepsy, frontal lobe epilepsies, supplementary motor epilepsies, and epilepsies of the motor cortex (Commission on Classification and Terminology of the International League Against Epilepsy, 1989).

Individuals with epilepsy are commonly considered to be at greater risk than the general population for MVCs (Krumholz, 1994; Taylor et al., 1996). The increased risk is thought to be due to a possible sudden loss of consciousness while driving and/or the propensity for anticonvulsant medications to impact cognition in the areas of concentration and reaction time. Although the supposition that individuals with epilepsy may be prone to MVCs due to side effects of medication is ever present in the literature on epilepsy and driving, there has been minimal investigation of the effects of anticonvulsant medications on driving behaviors. Rather, research efforts devoted to the investigation of epilepsy and driving have focused on reviewing laws regulating driving for persons with epilepsy, establishing a rate of MVCs for the population of drivers who suffer from epilepsy, and determining risk factors for MVCs in epilepsy.

DRIVING REGULATIONS

In order to prevent driving accidents and violations, statutes regarding physician reporting of patients with epilepsy to the driving authorities and revocation of driving privileges for individuals with uncontrolled seizures have been established. A person's seizures are considered controlled when a seizure free interval has elapsed. The required length of the seizure free interval varies across locales and ranges from 3 to 24 months. As such, state regulations of driving for individuals who suffer from epilepsy diverge widely. For a summary of the individual state laws on the requirement to report at-risk drivers with epilepsy and the information that must be provided to the respective Departments of Motor Vehicles see Krumholz (1994). Krauss et al. (2001) provided an updated summary of the individual state laws regarding driving restrictions, unpublished regulatory practices, and the role of physicians in judging driving safety of individuals with epilepsy.

On an international level, driving regulations for individuals with epilepsy vary as well, which creates difficulties for individuals with epilepsy who wish to drive while traveling abroad. The Joint Commission on Drivers' Licensing of the International Bureau for Epilepsy and the International League Against Epilepsy publicized summaries of the driving regulations in several countries and the responsibility of physicians to report individuals with epilepsy to the driving authorities across various nationalities (Parsonage et al., 1992). The regulations vary widely across nations and are too extensive to be reported within the body of this chapter. For a summary of the national regulations, see Fisher et al. (1994). Ooi and Gutrecht (2000) presented driving regulations for individuals with epilepsy and physician-reporting requirements from several previously unreported countries. Ooi and Gutrecht point out that due to mounting evidence that seizures can be controlled, the number of laws barring people with epilepsy from driving altogether has decreased and the requirement of a seizure free interval prior to obtaining permission to drive has been shortened. Countries have started to shift toward a more individualized approach when setting up laws with respect to drivers who have epilepsy.

Several authors have expanded upon the driving regulations in individual countries. For instance, Bener et al. (1996) reported that at the time of their article submission, there were no driving restrictions for individuals with epilepsy in the United Arab Emirates. Black and Lai (1997) provided a summary of the laws related to driving in individuals with epilepsy in South Australia. For a historical overview, and current status, of British regulations of driving in the epilepsy population see Taylor et al. (1996).

RATE OF DRIVING DIFFICULTIES

Some of the variability in national regulations for drivers with epilepsy may be due to the different rates of driving difficulties in drivers with epilepsy reported across these nationalities. Bener et al. (1996) reported that in the United Arab Emirates licensed drivers with epilepsy exhibited a significantly higher risk for property damage and traffic violations than the risk exhibited by licensed drivers without epilepsy. There was no difference between the two groups in rates of careless driving, speed violations, alcohol- and drug-related accidents. This information was collected from serial drivers treated in the "Accident Emergency Department" who responded to questionnaires and from their medical records. A study conducted in Denmark using a historical cohort register design found a risk factor for treatment at the casualty department after MVC that was increased seven-fold amongst individuals with epilepsy relative to matched healthy controls (Lings, 2001). The two subject groups were matched for age, gender, place of residence, and amount of time studied. The relevant time window was based on the index group and included the time period following diagnosis when the participant held a valid driver's license. Information was obtained on matched healthy controls for the same time period. All information for the study was obtained from official records.

Prior to the study conducted by Lings in 2001 a limited number of epidemiological studies had been performed studying rates of MVCs in the epilepsy population. As reviewed by Lings, early studies reported 1.3–1.95 increased relative risks for MVCs in individuals with epilepsy relative to controls. Given the limited number of these epidemiological studies more generally, it is unfortunate that the number of MVCs for the control groups and the incidence of diseases other than epilepsy amongst the healthy controls were not thoroughly investigated. Although the rates for MVC risk differ in the epidemiological studies, there is agreement across studies that risk for MVC is increased in individuals with epilepsy relative to healthy controls.

Studies using methodology other than the epidemiological approach to address the issue of driving behavior in epilepsy have generated findings discrepant with those reported in the epidemiological studies. For example, Taylor et al. (1996) conducted a 3-year retrospective study comparing rates of

MVCs, MVCs causing injury, and MVCs causing serious injury across drivers with epilepsy and healthy controls. Information was gathered from survey completion and statistical analyses controlled for age, gender, driving experience, and mileage across populations. While there was no increased risk for MVCs seen in the epilepsy sample, relative to healthy controls, a 40% increased risk was seen for serious injury and a two-fold increased risk rate for non-driver fatality in drivers with epilepsy relative to healthy controls. Other investigations that rely on self-report data for frequency of accidents and have compared index groups to general accident statistics for the population or accident referents have reported few differences in the rates of accidents between individuals with epilepsy and control groups (Taylor et al., 1995; Gislason et al., 1997).

More recently, researchers have begun to focus on driving behaviors across the different forms of epilepsy. Manji and Plant (2000) directed their efforts toward specific factors associated with temporal lobe epilepsy. As a result of the surgical procedure used to treat temporal lobe epilepsy, individuals frequently develop visual field cuts. Driving authorities have instituted requirements for minimal field of vision necessary to obtain or maintain a driver's license. These regulations, as well as the methods used for visual field assessment, vary across locations. Using the British guidelines for visual field criteria, one quarter of the sample of patients who had undergone the surgical procedure to correct for temporal lobe epilepsy exhibited visual field defects large enough to warrant license revocation. This raises a quality of life issue that should be addressed when considering treatment options, namely that while the surgical procedure may render individuals seizure free, it may also make them ineligible to drive. Berg et al. (2000) concentrated their driving research on refractory localization-related epilepsy (i.e., individuals with uncontrolled seizures that do not respond to pharmacological treatment). These individuals are generally restricted from operating motor vehicles, as they do not meet the required length for seizure free intervals. Based on review of medical records and self-report, 31.3% of the individuals with uncontrolled epilepsy had driven within the year prior to collection of data. Factors associated with increased likelihood of driving included having a current valid driver's license, ever having a driver's license, male gender, relatively younger age, and the perception that one is not disabled. Possibly salient factors that were not considered in the statistical models include prior MVCs, use of medications, visual field deficits, and cognitive functions.

Another recent study that differentiated between different forms of epilepsy used a computerized measure of visuospatial and attention functions to compare the driving-related skills of individuals with epilepsy (including participants with temporal lobe epilepsy and idiopathic generalized epilepsy) and healthy controls (Barcs et al., 1997). The computerized test used had been validated as a measure of driving abilities via comparison with practical, behind-the-wheel driving tests. The test yielded performance indices for activity, speed, and quality. Overall, no differences in performance were observed between the individuals with idiopathic generalized epilepsy being treated with one medication and healthy controls. However, individuals who suffer from temporal lobe epilepsy, especially those who were being treated with more than one medication, exhibited impaired performance on several parameters of the computerized test relative to healthy controls. Given the lack of control for medication type(s) in this study, it is unclear whether the performance decrement observed can be explained by the differences between particular forms of epilepsy or the side effects of polypharmaceutical treatment.

Beaussart et al. (1997) have pointed out that using seizure free intervals as indicators for determining driving capability is questionable given the reliance on the veracity of the individual's report of seizure frequency and the possibility that seizures will recur despite the period of remission. It is also noteworthy that the rate of MVCs in individuals with controlled epilepsy is only slightly higher than the rates of MVCs in the general population. The rate of MVCs in epileptic drivers is similar to the rate of MVCs in populations with other medical conditions (diabetes and heart disease) whose driving abilities are not regulated (Waller, 1965; Hansotia & Broste, 1991). Finally, the rate for MVCs in epileptic drivers is lower than the rate reported for individuals with other risk factors, such as, substance use (Lings, 2001), alcohol abuse and young drivers (Taylor et al., 1996). Given the risk rates across populations, the stringency of driving regulations for individuals with epilepsy, relative to those suffering from other medical or substance use disorders, should be reconsidered by legislators.

RISK FACTORS FOR DRIVING DIFFICULTIES

Although regulations have been established in order to limit the automobile driving of individuals who are at greatest risk of having a seizure while they drive, minimal investigation has been directed at isolating the specific risk factors for seizure-related MVCs. Krauss et al. (1999) conducted a retrospective case control study, comparing drivers with epilepsy who had MVCs while experiencing a seizure to drivers with epilepsy who had not been involved in MVCs. Information was collected via chart review and interviews. Protective factors that were shown to decrease the odds of MVCs in individuals with epilepsy include long seizure free intervals (i.e., intervals greater than, or equal to, 12 months), reliable auras, few prior non-seizure-related MVCs, reduction in dosage of anticonvulsant medication, and change or discontinuation of antiepileptic medication. Taylor et al. (1996) found two factors that protected against the increased rate for driving difficulties in drivers with epilepsy relative to healthy controls: antiepileptic medications and a seizure free interval of at least 3 years in duration. Interestingly, the presence of reliable auras was not shown to minimize accident risk.

SUMMARY AND LIMITATIONS OF RESEARCH ON
DRIVING AND EPILEPSY

A significant portion of the literature devoted to driving and epilepsy addresses the laws established to minimize negative driving outcomes for this population. Regulations of driving for individuals with epilepsy vary across location but are universally shifting toward shorter requirements for seizure free intervals and more individualized approaches. Although these laws are based on data that individuals with epilepsy show a higher rate of MVCs than healthy controls, some studies do not support this increased rate and also indicate that the rate of driving difficulties amongst people with epilepsy is similar to the rates for other medical populations whose driving is not regulated by the law (see Table 8.2). Some protective factors, including long seizure free intervals and the proper usage of anticonvulsant medications, have been identified for minimizing driving difficulties in individuals with epilepsy.

Limitations of studies investigating driving behavior amongst individuals with epilepsy include the small, non-representative samples that rarely address the different forms of epilepsy, inadequate control groups and lack of reliable data on MVCs. Reliance on medical records to obtain information on driving difficulties introduces a potential confound; the possibility that individuals with epilepsy seek medical treatment more or less frequently than healthy controls due to their familiarity with the medical system or their concerns over having their licenses revoked. Another confounding factor that is frequently neglected in studies of driving behavior and epilepsy is the difference between epileptic drivers and healthy control drivers in actual miles driven. The dependent measures used in these studies are not uniform making comparisons across studies difficult. Interestingly, studies of the relationship between cognitive difficulties and driving skills in individuals with epilepsy are not present in the literature. The Joint Commission on Drivers' Licensing of the International Bureau for Epilepsy and the International League Against Epilepsy did not include a

TABLE 8.2   Comparison of Epileptic and Control Drivers Using Relative Risk Ratios.

Study	MVC	MVC causing injury	MVC causing serious injury	Driving offenses
Waller (1965)	1.95	–	–	–
Crancer et al. (1968)	1.3	–	–	–
Taylor et al. (1996)	0.77	1.08	1.33	–
Hansiota et al. (1991)	1.33	1.57	–	–
Bener et al. (1996)	–	–	–	1.91
Lings (2001)	7.07	–	–	–

– = Not assessed.

recommendation for assessment of cognition in its guidelines for determining fitness to drive an automobile. Given the knowledge from other medical populations that cognitive factors affect driving performance, and the fact that many individuals with epilepsy suffer from cognitive impairment, this omission is troubling. Future research on driving skills in epilepsy should address cognitive abilities, both with respect to disease factors and the effects of anticonvulsant medications.

PSYCHIATRIC DISORDERS

When attempting to identify problem drivers, people who suffer from psychiatric disorders have traditionally been viewed as "accident-prone" (Niveau & Kelley-Puskas, 2001). Potential problems relevant to driving that are present amongst individuals with psychiatric disorders include medication effects, degree of alcohol consumption and substance use, driving inexperience, anxiety, difficulty responding to stressful situations, and medical comorbidity. Additionally, the Federal Highway Administration Conference on psychiatric disorders identified specific areas of cognitive impairment associated with psychiatric disorders that may impact driving ability, including attention, concentration, memory, information processing ability, visuospatial functions, motor response latency, impulse control, judgment, and problem solving (Metzner et al., 1993). However, the impact of impaired cognition on driving abilities has been minimally investigated in the population of individuals with psychiatric illness. Furthermore, a direct relationship between severity of psychiatric illness and functional driving incapacity has yet to be established (Metzner et al., 1993). Numerous confounds, such as the effects of psychotropic medications (which will be addressed in this chapter), may impact on the posited relationship between psychiatric disorders and driving skills. Although a significant literature exists concerning MVCs and psychiatric illness, the body of work reveals limited and inconclusive empirical findings due to, in part, a lack of control for confounding variables (Metzner et al., 1993). This section of the chapter will review the early research on rates of MVCs in people with psychiatric disorders and the responsibility of psychiatrists to assess driving fitness in this population. Because of the nature of the research conducted, the majority of this discussion of driving and psychiatric disorders will focus on the effects of psychotropic medications on driving ability.

DRIVING RISK IN PSYCHIATRIC POPULATIONS

Early research on driving ability and psychiatric disorders indicated that psychiatric patients as a whole do not present a greater risk for MVCs than the general population (Buttiglieri & Guenette, 1967), excluding comorbidity with alcohol and substance use disorders (Maki & Linnoila, 1976; Armstrong & Whitlock, 1980). However, certain types of psychopathology were shown to have higher accident rates than the general population, such as personality or psychoneurotic disorders (Crancer & Quiring, 1969; Tsuang et al., 1985). With regard to psychotic disorders, individuals with schizophrenia were reported to drive less than matched healthy controls and have more accidents per mile driven based on self-report (Edlund et al., 1989). Similarly, earlier research reported a two-fold incidence of traffic accidents per mile driven in outpatient schizophrenics relative to control subjects (Waller, 1965). Following the early investigations of rates of negative driving behaviors in psychiatric disorders, researchers began to focus efforts on other aspects of driving in this population, that is, driving regulations, psychiatric consequences of MVCs and the effects of psychotropic medications on driving across various psychiatric disorders.

DRIVING REGULATIONS

A recent resurgence in the research of driving practices and psychiatric disorders has occurred due to legal concerns regarding the responsibility of psychiatrists toward patients who may not be fit to drive. Early research had demonstrated that certain types of psychopathology might place an individual at a higher risk for negative driving behaviors than healthy controls. Local laws addressing this issue and the statutes set up to prevent driving accidents and violations due to patients' psychiatric disorders vary considerably. Given the wide range of statutes, a review of the laws is beyond the scope of this chapter. For a summary of the individual state laws on the requirement to report at-risk drivers and what type of information must be provided to the respective Departments of Motor Vehicles see Metzner et al. (1993). Morgan (1998) provides a summary of the British guidelines from the Driver and Vehicle Licensing Agency, as well as the British General Medical Council.

Although physicians are required in certain locales to report individuals with psychiatric disorders to the driving authorities, the efficacy of this method of accident prevention was not addressed prior to establishment of the statutes. Niveau and Kelley-Puskas (2001) attempted to ascertain whether this mode of traffic accident prevention is efficacious. They compared drivers who had been reported to driving authorities due to psychiatric illness (index group) and drivers whose licenses were revoked due to the presence of a psychiatric disorder at the time of an MVC or driving violation (control group). Retrospective data were collected for the time period prior to the index group being reported to the driving authorities and prior to the revocation of the control group's driver licenses. Sociodemographic and medical information, as well as driving records from the local bureau of motor vehicles and results of psychiatric evaluations were collected for each participant. Relative to the control group, participants in the index group exhibited more severe psychiatric conditions. However, in contrast to expectations, the index group participants had fewer driving accidents and violations on their driving records than controls had. These data suggest that individuals who are deemed incapable of driving due to psychiatric illness by their psychiatrists may not represent the subgroup of mentally ill individuals at highest risk for unsafe driving behaviors (Niveau & Kelley-Puskas, 2001).

PSYCHIATRIC CONSEQUENCES OF MVCS

Investigations in the area of psychiatric disorders and driving also extend to psychiatric consequences of motor vehicle collisions. Psychological and psychiatric sequelae of automobile accidents were little studied until the late 1980s, at which point the majority of research was conducted outside the United States and primarily employed survey methods. After reviewing the literature on psychiatric consequences of MVCs, Blanchard et al. (1995) reported that the percentage of MVC victims who develop Post-Traumatic Stress Disorder (PTSD) subsequent to their MVCs varies widely, ranging from 1 to 100% in treatment seeking samples and from 8 to 46% in non-treatment seeking populations. Comorbid diagnoses developed post-MVC included other anxiety disorders and mood disorders, especially driving phobias and major depression. Blanchard et al. (1995) critiqued the literature on psychiatric consequences of MVCs stating that studies utilized clinical, rather than structured, interview methods, referral sources varied widely across samples, and that time post MVC fluctuated greatly for study participants.

An early prospective study examining the psychiatric consequences of MVCs followed consecutive MVC victims who visited the hospital emergency room for a period of one year following their MVC. Data was collected via interviews, rating scales, medical charts, and police and ambulance reports. One quarter of the MVC victims described psychiatric symptoms at one-year follow-up. Patterns of psychiatric symptomatology seen at outcome were categorized as general emotional distress, phobic anxiety and PTSD. Premorbid psychiatric problems reported by the MVC victims were shown to contribute to psychiatric outcome one-year post-MVC. Given the absence of a control group, the presence of confounding factors such as traumatic brain injuries and injury severity, and the minimal information on premorbid psychiatric status, suggest that these findings must be interpreted with caution (Mayou et al., 1993).

Blanchard et al. (1994, 1995) conducted further research into psychiatric morbidity following road traffic accidents. Psychiatric symptomatology, prior traumatic experiences, and driving behaviors of individuals who had recently experienced MVCs and sought medical attention were compared to those of a non-MVC control group. Information was collected via structured and clinical interviews, as well as rating scales. Of the MVC group, following their motor vehicle collision, 46% exhibited PTSD and 100% exhibited some level of driving avoidance, relative to a rate of 2.5% of the controls that exhibited PTSD. Driving avoidance was not assessed in the control group. The MVC participants had experienced significantly more prior traumatic experiences (including prior motor vehicle collisions as well as other traumas), and tended to exhibit more lifetime Axis-I diagnoses (such as mood and anxiety disorders), relative to the control participants

(Blanchard et al., 1994). These findings were replicated in a larger sample (Blanchard et al., 1995). Further randomization of the MVC victim sample, and information on pre-MVC psychiatric status obtained via sources other than the proband, would improve upon this study design. Clearly, implementation of more scientifically rigorous studies is necessary in this area, in order to provide direction for psychological intervention following traffic accidents.

PSYCHOTROPIC MEDICATIONS

While psychoactive medications are generally thought to affect driving behavior and may complicate the relationship between psychiatric disorders and driving skills, investigators disagree as to whether the medications yield positive or negative effects on driving performance. These medications have the potential to impair driving ability due to sedation and/or motor difficulties resulting from treatment and their capacity to potentiate the effects of alcohol, sedatives, hypnotics, narcotics, and antihistamines. On the other hand, psychotropic medications may enhance driving by increasing concentration and improving judgment. Factors that should be addressed when conducting research on the effects of psychoactive medications on driving behaviors include the differential effects of chronic versus acute administration, the influence of the psychiatric disorder itself on driving behavior, and difficulty establishing valid laboratory tests of driving behavior.

ANTIPSYCHOTIC MEDICATIONS

According to a review of the literature published in 1985, the majority of studies reported that acute administration of antipsychotics to healthy controls caused impairment on tests of psychomotor performance. Some of these skills, such as visual–motor coordination, can be extrapolated to driving performance. However, whereas acute administration of antipsychotic medication to a healthy control engenders sedation and decreased alertness, these side effects are diminished with chronic administration in a clinical population. Furthermore, persons with schizophrenia exhibit improvement on psychomotor tests during chronic treatment with antipsychotic agents. Thus, although acute administration of antipsychotics to healthy controls results in impaired driving behavior, it is possible that chronic administration of antipsychotics may enhance driving behavior for schizophrenic individuals. It was clear that further research into the effects of chronic administration of antipsychotics to schizophrenics on driving behavior, driving behaviors in unmedicated persons with schizophrenia, and the differential effects on driving behavior of the sedating and non-sedating antipsychotics was needed.

Bech (1975) compared the performance of hospital inpatients with and without psychotic symptoms on a driving simulator pre- and post-treatment with antipsychotic medications. The two groups differed in baseline driving-related performance, such that the psychotic group had prolonged brake time and their performance deteriorated more markedly over trials. Following pharmacological treatment, enhanced performance was seen in the psychotic group, but was not observed in the non-psychotic group. Diagnoses, ongoing pharmacological treatment, and length of treatment varied widely for study participants. Although the results of this study are important, the lack of standardization in variables central to this research limits the generalizability of these findings.

Recent investigations of the effect of antipsychotic medications on driving have attempted to be more scientifically rigorous. Wylie et al. (1993) compared the performance of medicated, stable, and non-psychotic schizophrenics to the performance of unmedicated healthy controls on a simulated driving test. Schizophrenic participants were being treated with one of two possible depot neuroleptics and were excluded from participation if they were receiving any other regular medication. Steering accuracy, brake reaction time, and number of non-responses to red lights were used as indices of performance on the driving simulator. Persons with schizophrenia performed significantly worse than the control group on all driving indices. Similarly, Grabe et al. (1999) compared the psychomotor abilities of schizophrenic inpatients being treated with clozapine to those being treated with typical neuroleptics. The psychomotor test used targeted reaction time, vigilance, visual perception and stress tolerance and has been well correlated with actual behind-the-wheel driving performance. While the authors hypothesized that the clozapine treatment group would be less impaired due to the absence of sedating side effects, both subject groups were equally impaired on the psychomotor test. Unfortunately, due to the lack of a no-medication control group, it is unclear whether these effects are related specifically to schizophrenia (e.g., cognitive dysfunction) or some general medication effect. Psychiatric comorbidity, medication types (excluding the clozapine group), and medication dosages remain uncontrolled in many such studies. Assessment of the separate contributions of schizophrenia and antipsychotic medications to driving performance is still lacking.

ANTI-ANXIETY MEDICATIONS

Benzodiazepines, the most widely prescribed class of antianxiety medications, may impact driving behavior due to their side effects of sedation, increased drowsiness, and disinhibition. A double-blind crossover trial of medazepam was conducted in an inpatient group diagnosed with anxiety disorders (Moore, 1977). Results showed that among the participants, performance on a test of braking and on a driving simulation was at the same level irrespective of agent administered (i.e., medazepam or placebo). However, performance on a behind-the-wheel evaluation following medazepam administration included significantly more technical (or minor) errors than performance post-placebo administration. There were no differences in the number of dangerous (or major) driving errors made in the placebo and medazepam conditions. The driving examiners were unaware of which participants were receiving the active drug or placebo. As medazepam was administered below therapeutic levels in this study, generalization to actual clinical samples should be done with caution.

The effect of an alternate benzodiazepine, diazepam, on driving behavior was studied in a group of anxiety disordered outpatient participants (van Laar et al., 1992). Following a baseline week of placebo administration, diazepam was administered during a double-blind drug treatment period of 4 weeks. Participants completed a behind-the-wheel driving evaluation during the baseline week and each of the four treatment weeks. Driving was measured through speed and lateral position of the vehicle. Relative to performance in the placebo condition, lateral vehicle positioning was impaired during the first 3 weeks of diazepam administration and speed control was impaired during the first week of diazepam administration. During the drug treatment weeks when impairment on either lateral vehicle positioning or speed control was not observed, performance level was similar to baseline and was not indicative of improvement. Due to small sample size ($n = 12$), it was not possible to explore the predictors of driving impairment during treatment with benzodiazepines in this study.

In a similar report of three studies where benzodiazepine and benzodiazepine-like anxiolytics were administered in double-blind placebo controlled studies to either individuals diagnosed with anxiety disorders or healthy controls, the medications produced marked and pervasive driving impairment on two forms of behind-the-wheel evaluations (O'Hanlon et al., 1995). It is noteworthy that no significant differences were seen between healthy control and anxious individuals' performance in the baseline or drug conditions, suggesting that it is the medication and not a component of the psychiatric disorder that is affecting driving behavior in this case. However, these clinical trials were only continued for a week of medication administration and thus may not represent actual driving performance during chronic administration of anxiolytic agents. Studies using larger sample sizes, longer medication trials, therapeutic levels of medication, as well as controlling for comorbidity, medication type and medication dosing are still necessary to allow for reliable and valid conclusions regarding the effects of psychoactive medications on driving behavior.

PSYCHIATRIC DISORDERS: SUMMARY AND CONCLUSIONS

Early investigations of driving skills amongst individuals with psychiatric disorders generated inconclusive findings regarding risk for MVC that differed across studies and depending on the diagnostic group being investigated. More recent research focused on physician responsibility to assess their patients' driving fitness. As of yet, there is no clear evidence that physicians are successful in determining which individuals suffering from psychiatric disorders are at greatest risk for negative driving outcomes. Considerable data suggest that some portion of MVC victims exhibits psychiatric symptomatology following the incident. However, the risk factors that predispose individuals to developing psychiatric illness following MVCs remain unclear. The majority of the studies in the area of psychiatric disorders and driving ability address the effects of psychotropic medications while other factors central to understanding the relationship between psychiatric disorders and driving risk have received minimal attention.

Taken as a whole, the body of research on psychiatric disorders and driving difficulties is inconclusive due to the presence of myriad confounding factors and faulty empirical designs. Psychiatric dysfunction is not a unitary construct and rigorous controls need to be implemented in order to tease apart the contributions of relevant factors, such as medication effects versus disease factors. Rather than devoting further efforts to determining the rates of driving difficulties amongst the psychiatric population as a whole, efforts should be directed toward establishing the differential susceptibility toward negative driving behaviors across different psychiatric conditions. Once the psychiatric disorders that are at highest risk for negative driving outcomes have been identified, assessment of possible contributing factors, such as medication effects, physical disabilities, and cognition should be conducted. Although the Federal Highway Administration Conference on psychiatric disorders identified specific areas of cognitive impairment associated with psychiatric disorders that may impact driving ability in 1991, to date these cognitive constructs have not been investigated with regard to driving ability and psychiatric disorders.

CONCLUSIONS

The ability to operate a motor vehicle is a complex behavior that compromises physical, visual, and cognitive functions. This chapter has presented a review of the driving literature for four medical conditions where the aforementioned functions may be impaired, potentially impacting driving behaviors. Across the four conditions, researchers have investigated the rates of driving difficulties, the risks for problematic driving behaviors, and the regulations governing driving for the particular population. The depth of the driving literature and the sophistication of methodology vary across the four conditions.

Despite the wide range of investigations conducted, there are some similarities in the driving literature across the four conditions reviewed in this chapter that should be noted. Firstly, while cognition has been demonstrated to be an integral component of driving ability, assessment of cognitive factors has not played a fundamental role in research of driving skills across these populations with neurological and psychiatric disorders. Interestingly, for the two populations (MS and ADHD) where driving research has been a recent addition to conceptualization of complex behaviors impacted by the disorder, early investigations into the relationship between cognitive functioning and driving abilities have been conducted. On the other hand, for those disorders (i.e., epilepsy and psychiatric conditions), where investigations into driving capacity have been conducted for some time, little to no research into the impact of impaired cognition on driving skills has been conducted. Empirical investigations of how the cognitive features of these conditions affect driving ability is necessary to determine which specific cognitive factors are associated with risks in driving behavior. Research has yet to advance beyond the suggestion of which cognitive functions may be associated with poor driving in each condition (see Table 8.3). Furthermore, regarding clinical practice, determination of driving capacity following neurological compromise typically does not involve assessment of cognitive functions. The clinical community has yet to reach agreement on a standard procedure for assessment of driving abilities in most situations. Potentially unsafe drivers should be assessed carefully through medical and neuropsychological examinations that evaluate physical, visual, and cognitive prerequisite functions for motor vehicle operation.

A second commonality present in the driving literature across the four conditions presented in this chapter is the variability across studies in the selection of dependent measures. Measures used include self-report of driving behaviors via rating scales and interviews, review of medical and motor vehicle department records, and performance on tests of driving knowledge and skill, including driving simulators and computerized measures. The subjective nature of self-report and the incomplete picture obtained when relying upon a single dependent measure make the generalizability of the findings of some studies difficult to interpret. Even among more quantitative measures, the divergent methodology across studies makes comparison of results difficult. It is recommended that attention

TABLE 8.3   Suggested Cognitive Contributors to Driving Difficulties Across Conditions.

Cognitive construct	ADHD	MS	Psychiatric disorders	Epilepsy
Attention	✓	✓	✓	✓
Executive functions	✓	✓		
Impulse control	✓		✓	
Information processing			✓	
Judgment			✓	
Memory			✓	
Motor response latency			✓	
Problem solving			✓	
Processing speed		✓		
Reaction time				✓
Visuoperceptual skills		✓	✓	

be directed toward the development of statistically reliable and valid measures of driving behaviors that can be applied across participant populations.

A final common feature in the driving literature across the four conditions is the presence of myriad confounding factors. Numerous conditions that are shown to impact on driving behavior and have not been rigorously controlled or investigated in these studies include gender, degree of driving experience, comorbid symptomatology, medication, and treatment effects. Development of efficacious clinical evaluations of driving behavior and interventions to improve driving skills depends on improvement of this body of research.

REFERENCES

American Psychiatric Association (1994). *Diagnostic and Statistical Manual of Mental Disorders* (4th ed). Washington DC: Author.

Armstrong, J. L., & Whitlock, F. A. (1980). Mental illness and road traffic accidents. *Aust. NZ. J. Psychiatr., 14*, 53–60.

Barcs, G., Vitrai, J., & Halasz, P. (1997). Investigation of vehicle driving ability in two diagnostic groups of epileptic patients with special neuropsychological approach. *Med. Law., 16*, 277–287.

Barkley, R. A. (1997). Behavioral inhibition, sustained attention, and executive functions: constructing a unifying theory of ADHD. *Psychol. Bull., 121*, 65–94.

Barkley, R. A., Murphy, K. R., DuPaul, G. I., Bush, T. (2002). Driving in young adults with attention deficit hyperactivity disorder: Knowledge, performance, adverse outcomes, and the role of executive functioning. *J Int Neuropsychol Soc, 8*, 655–672.

Barkley, R. A., Guevremont, D. C., Anastopoulos, A. D., DuPaul, G. J., & Shelton, T. L. (1993). Driving-related risks and outcomes of attention deficit hyperactivity disorder in adolescents and young adults: A 3- to 5-year follow-up survey. *Pediatrics, 92*, 212–218.

Barkley, R. A., Murphy, K. R., & Kwasnik, D. (1996). Motor vehicle driving competencies and risks in teens and young adults with attention deficit hyperactivity disorder. *Pediatrics, 98*, 1089–1095.

Beaussart, M., Beaussart-Defaye, J., Lamiaux, J. M., & Grubar, J. C. (1997). Epileptic drivers – a study of 1,089 patients. *Med. Law., 16*, 295–306.

Bech, P. (1975). Mental illness and simulated driving: Before and during treatment. *Pharmakopsychiatr. Neuropsychopharmakol., 8*, 143–150.

Bener, A., Murdoch, J. C., Achan, N. V., Karama, A. H., & Sztriha, L. (1996). The effect of epilepsy on road traffic accidents and casualties. *Seizure, 5*, 215–219.

Berg, A. T., Vickrey, B. G., Sperling, M. R. et al. (2000). Driving in adults with refractory localization-related epilepsy. Multi-Center Study of Epilepsy Surgery. *Neurology, 54*, 625–630.

Bitsch, A., Schuchardt, J., Bunkowski, S., Kuhlmann, T., & Bruck, W. (2000). Acute axonal injury in multiple sclerosis. Correlation with demyelination and inflammation. *Brain, 123*(Pt 6), 1174–1183.

Black, A. B., & Lai, N. Y. (1997). Epilepsy and driving in South Australia – an assessment of compulsory notification. *Med. Law., 16*, 253–267.

Blanchard, E. B., Hickling, E. J., Taylor, A. E., Loos, W. R., & Gerardi, R. J. (1994). Psychological morbidity associated with motor vehicle accidents. *Behav Res Ther., 32*, 283–290.

Blanchard, E. B., Hickling, E. J., Taylor, A. E., & Loos, W. (1995). Psychiatric morbidity associated with motor vehicle accidents. *J. Nerv. Ment. Dis., 183*, 495–504.

Buttiglieri, M. W., & Guenette, M. (1967). Driving record of neuropsychiatric patients. *J. Appl. Psychol., 51*, 96–100.

Commission on Classification and Terminology of the International League Against Epilepsy (1989). Proposal for revised classification of epilepsies and epileptic syndromes. *Epilepsia, 30*, 389–399.

Cox, D. J., Merkel, R. L., Kovatchev, B., & Seward, R. (2000). Effect of stimulant medication on driving performance of young adults with attention-deficit hyperactivity disorder: A preliminary double-blind placebo controlled trial. *J. Nerv. Ment. Dis.*, *188*, 230–234.

Crancer, A., & McMurray, L. (1968). Accident and violation rates of Washington's medically restricted drivers. *JAMA*, *205*, 74–78.

Crancer, A. Jr., & Quiring, D. L. (1969). The mentally ill as motor vehicle operators. *Am. J. Psychiatr.*, *126*, 807–813.

DeLuca, J., Barbieri-Berger, S., & Johnson, S. K. (1994). The nature of memory impairments in multiple sclerosis: Acquisition versus retrieval. *J. Clin. Exp. Neuropsychol.*, *16*, 183–189.

DeLuca, J., Gaudino, E. A., Diamond, B. J., Christodoulou, C., & Engel, R. A. (1998). Acquisition and storage deficits in multiple sclerosis. *J. Clin. Exp. Neuropsychol.*, *20*, 376–390.

Devinsky, O. (1994). Seizure disorders. *Clin. Symp.*, *46*, 2–34.

Douglas, V. I. (1983). Attentional and cognitive problems. In: M. Rutter (Ed.), *Developmental Neuropsychiatry* (pp. 280–329). New York: Guilford Press.

National Highway Traffic Safety Administration (1997). Driving histories of ADHD. *Ann. Emerg. Med.*, *29*, 546–547. Discussion 547-8.

Edlund, M. J., Conrad, C., & Morris, P. (1989). Accidents among schizophrenic outpatients. *Compr. Psychiatr.*, *30*, 522–526.

Fisher, R. S., Parsonage, M., Beaussart, M. et al. (1994). Epilepsy and driving: an international perspective. Joint Commission on Drivers' Licensing of the International Bureau for Epilepsy and the International League Against Epilepsy. *Epilepsia*, *35*, 675–684.

Gislason, T., Tomasson, K., Reynisdottir, H., Bjornsson, J. K., & Kristbjarnarson, H. (1997). Medical risk factors amongst drivers in single-car accidents. *J. Intern. Med.*, *241*, 213–219.

Goodwill, C. J. (1984). Mobility for the disabled patient. *Int. Rehabil. Med.*, *6*, iii–iv.

Grabe, H. J., Wolf, T., Gratz, S., & Laux, G. (1999). The influence of clozapine and typical neuroleptics on information processing of the central nervous system under clinical conditions in schizophrenic disorders: Implications for fitness to drive. *Neuropsychobiology*, *40* 196–201.

Hansotia, P., & Broste, S. K. (1991). The effect of epilepsy or diabetes mellitus on the risk of automobile accidents. *N. Engl. J. Med.*, *324*, 22–26.

Hechtman, L., & Weiss, G. (1986). Controlled prospective fifteen year follow-up of hyperactives as adults: Non-medical drug and alcohol use and anti-social behaviour. *Can. J. Psychiatr.*, *31*, 557–567.

Knecht, J. (1977). [The multiple sclerosis patient as a driver]. *Schweiz Med Wochenschr*, *107*, 373–378.

Krauss, G. L., Krumholz, A., Carter, R. C., Li, G., & Kaplan, P. (1999). Risk factors for seizure-related motor vehicle crashes in patients with epilepsy. *Neurology*, *52*, 1324–1329.

Krauss, G. L., Ampaw, L., & Krumholz, A. (2001). Individual state driving restrictions for people with epilepsy in the US. *Neurology*, *57*, 1780–1785.

Krumholz, A. (1994). Driving and epilepsy: A historical perspective and review of current regulations. *Epilepsia*, *35*, 668–674.

Lapham, S. C., Smith, E., C'de Baca, J. et al. (2001). Prevalence of psychiatric disorders among persons convicted of driving while impaired. *Arch. Gen. Psychiatr.*, *58*, 943–949.

Lings, S. (2001). Increased driving accident frequency in Danish patients with epilepsy. *Neurology*, *57*, 435–439.

Maki, M., & Linnoila, M. (1976). Characteristics of driving in relation to the drug and alcohol use of Finnish outpatients. *Mod. Probl. Pharmacopsychiatr.*, *11*, 11–21.

Manji, H., & Plant, G. T. (2000). Epilepsy surgery, visual fields, and driving: A study of the visual field criteria for driving in patients after temporal lobe epilepsy surgery with a comparison of Goldmann and Esterman perimetry. *J. Neurol. Neurosurg. Psychiatr.*, *68*, 80–82.

Marks, D. J., Newcorn, J. H., & Halperin, J. M. (2001). Comorbidity in adults with attention-deficit/hyperactivity disorder. *Ann. NY. Acad. Sci.*, *931*, 216–238.

Mayou, R., Bryant, B., & Duthie, R. (1993). Psychiatric consequences of road traffic accidents. *BMJ*, *307*, 647–651.

Metzner, J. L., Dentino, A. N., Godard, S. L., Hay, D. P., Hay, L., & Linnoila, M. (1993). Impairment in driving and psychiatric illness. *J. Neuropsychiatr. Clin. Neurosci.*, *5*, 211–220.

Michon, J. A. (1985). A critical review of driver behavior models: What we know, what should we do?. In: L. Evans, & R. Schwing (Eds.), *Human Behavior and Traffic Safety*. New York: Plenum Press.

Miller, A. (2001). Clinical features. In: D. S. Cook (Ed.), *Handbook of Multiple Sclerosis* (3rd ed.) (pp. 213–232). New York: Marcel Dekker.

Minden, S. L., & Schiffer, R. B. (1990). Affective disorders in multiple sclerosis. Review and recommendations for clinical research. *Arch. Neurol.*, *47*, 98–104.

Moore, N. C. (1977). Medazepam and the driving ability of anxious patients. *Psychopharmacology (Berl).*, *52*, 103–106.

Morgan, J. F. (1998). DVLA and GMC guidelines on "fitness to drive" and psychiatric disorders: Knowledge following an educational campaign. *Med. Sci. Law.*, *38*, 28–33.

Murphy, K., & Barkley, R. A. (1996). Attention deficit hyperactivity disorder adults: Comorbidities and adaptive impairments. *Compr. Psychiatr.*, *37*, 393–401.

Nada-Raja, S., Langley, J. D., McGee, R., Williams, S. M., Begg, D. J., & Reeder, A. I. (1997). Inattentive and hyperactive behaviors and driving offenses in adolescence. *J. Am. Acad. Child. Adolesc. Psychiatr.*, *36*, 515–522.

Neppe, V. M., & Tucker, G. J. (1988). Modern perspectives on epilepsy in relation to psychiatry: Classification and evaluation. *Hosp. Community Psychiatr.*, *39*, 263–271.

Niveau, G., & Kelley-Puskas, M. (2001). Psychiatric disorders and fitness to drive. *J. Med. Ethics.*, *27*, 36–39.

O'Hanlon, J. F., Vermeeren, A., Uiterwijk, M. M., van Veggel, L. M., & Swijgman, H. F. (1995). Anxiolytics' effects on the actual driving performance of patients and healthy volunteers in a standardized test. An integration of three studies. *Neuropsychobiology*, *31*, 81–88.

Ooi, W. W., & Gutrecht, J. A. (2000). International regulations for automobile driving and epilepsy. *J. Travel. Med.*, *7*, 1–4.

Parsonage, M., Beaussart, M., Baldin, P.F., et al. (1992). Epilepsy and driving license regulations. Report by the ILAE/IBE Commission on Drivers' Licensing. The Netherland: The International League Against Epilepsy and The International Bureau for Epilepsy.

Pryse-Phillips, W., & Costello, F. (2001). The epidemiology of multiple sclerosis. In: S. D. Cook (Ed.), *Handbook of Multiple Sclerosis* (3rd ed.) (pp. 15–33). New York: Marcel Dekker.

Rao, S. M. (1986). Neuropsychology of multiple sclerosis: A critical review. *J. Clin. Exp. Neuropsychol.*, *8*, 503–542.

Schanke, A. K., Grimsmo, J., & Sundet, K. (1995). [Multiple sclerosis and prerequisites for driver's licence. A retrospective study of 33 patients with multiple sclerosis assessed at Sunnaas hospital]. *Tidsskr Nor Laegeforen*, *115*, 1349–1352.

Schultheis, M. T., Garay, E., & DeLuca, J. (2001). The influence of cognitive impairment on driving performance in multiple sclerosis. *Neurology*, *56*, 1089–1094.

Schultheis, M.T., Garay, E., Millis, S.R., DeLuca, J. (2002). Motor vehicle crashes and violations among drivers with multiple sclerosis. *Arch. Phys. Med. Rehabil. 8*, 1175–8.

Schultheis, M. T., Hillary, F., & Chute, D. L. (2003). The Neurocognitive Driving Test: Applying technology to the assessment of driving ability following brain injury. *Rehabil. Psychol.*, *5*, 275–280.

Taylor, J., Chadwick, D. W., & Johnson, T. (1995). Accident experience and notification rates in people with recent seizures, epilepsy or undiagnosed episodes of loss of consciousness. *QJM*, *88*, 733–740.

Taylor, J., Chadwick, D., & Johnson, T. (1996). Risk of accidents in drivers with epilepsy. *J. Neurol. Neurosurg. Psychiatr.*, *60*, 621–627.

Trapp, B. D., Peterson, J., Ransohoff, R. M., Rudick, R., Mork, S., & Bo, L. (1998). Axonal transection in the lesions of multiple sclerosis. *N. Engl. J. Med.*, *338*, 278–285.

Tsuang, M. T., Boor, M., & Fleming, J. A. (1985). Psychiatric aspects of traffic accidents. *Am. J. Psychiatr.*, *142*, 538–546.

US Department of Education (1988). Youth indicators 1988: Trends in the well-being of American youth. Washington DC: US Government Printing Office, DE Publication No. 065-000-00347-3.

van Laar, M. W., Volkerts, E. R., & van Willigenburg, A. P. (1992). Therapeutic effects and effects on actual driving performance of chronically administered buspirone and diazepam in anxious outpatients. *J. Clin. Psychopharmacol.*, *12*, 86–95.

Waller, J. A. (1965). Chronic medical conditions and traffic safety: Review of the California experience. *N. Engl. J. Med.*, *273*, 1413–1420.

Woodward, L. J., Fergusson, D. M., & Horwood, L. J. (2000). Driving outcomes of young people with attentional difficulties in adolescence. *J. Am. Acad. Child. Adolesc. Psychiatr.*, *39*, 627–634.

Wylie, K. R., Thompson, D. J., & Wildgust, H. J. (1993). Effects of depot neuroleptics on driving performance in chronic schizophrenic patients. *J. Neurol. Neurosurg. Psychiatr.*, *56*, 910–913.

9

DRIVING, MEDICAL ILLNESS, AND MEDICATIONS

THOMAS GALSKI, LORAN VOCATURO AND THOMAS M. GALSKI

Mobility in general but driving in particular is an important part of every adults' life in American society. It is crucial to overall well-being, autonomy, independence, and self-sufficiency for individuals of all ages. In fact, it has been shown that cessation of driving can have profound effects on some people's lives, including changes in health, isolation, and depression (Legh-Smith et al., 1986; Marottoli et al., 1997; Fonda et al., 2001).

But driving is a demanding activity that requires the complex interaction of physical and cognitive skills and abilities. And any reduction or loss of abilities due to injury, illness or disease and/or the medical treatment of such conditions have the obvious potential to adversely affect a person's driving capacity and thereby increase the risk of accidents, including the risk of death and/or injury to self and others as well as property damage.

In the interest of preserving independence and autonomy of drivers and eliminating the risk of death and injury to drivers and others, President Hoover was an earlier figure in our society who called for a National Conference to uncover tasks necessary to safely operate an automobile; furthermore, he challenged scientists to define the parameters for driving and relate these parameters to probability of an accident. Since that time scientists and investigators, recognizing the importance of studying real-world driving, have attempted to identify specific skills and abilities regarded as important in safe driving, the extent to which each is necessary for operation of a motor vehicle and the relationship of abilities to accidents.

The charge is generally difficult and success in these endeavors has been slow at least in part because:

a. there are significant problems in establishing valid and reliable measures of driving performance. There are many tests used singly or in combination with others that are part of off-road and on-road methods to evaluate driving performance but no protocol has received general acceptance;

b. accidents and crashes, the common measure of real-world driving performance, are so relatively rare (affect only 10% of drivers per year and occur 1–2 times/100,00 miles of driving) that researchers and evaluators find themselves trying to predict an improbable event;

c. accidents have many causes, some of which may not be related to the driver, for example, weather, mechanical error.

Investigators looking at the relationship between driving, illness and disease are further hampered by limited availability of or access to study populations. While some medical conditions are common, such as diabetes, with a relatively large sample size of drivers available for study, sample sizes for other conditions, for example, drivers with dementia, are more problematic. Additionally, many individuals have co-morbidities and/or use various medications alone or in combination with others; these groups are difficult to collect for study in large sample sizes.

Moreover, medical illness and disease are typically regarded as conditions or disabilities resulting from end-organ dysfunction, such as a cardiac disorder, or metabolic deficiency, such as diabetes. This *medical model* fails to recognize the link between physiologic and functional capacity that is at the core of driving or consider the net effect of all physiological and pathological forces acting on drivers at the same time (Nagi, 1976; Retchin, 1989). Consequently, driving may tend to be viewed in terms of the medical conditions or diagnoses per se rather than a driver's level of functional ability in driving (Waller, 1965; Fitten et al., 1996).

Nevertheless, there has been a number of studies in recent decades that attempted to examine the relationship between medical conditions, medications and the measurement of driving performance. The following review provides a look into this relationship in an effort to convey researchers' areas of interest, the types of studies and methodologies, and findings in terms of the most commonly used measure of safety, that is, accidents, crashes, traffic violations.

MEDICAL CONDITIONS

CARDIOVASCULAR DISEASES AND DISORDERS

The relationship between driving performance and a number of cardiovascular diseases and disorders, including heart disease, myocardial infarction, arrhythmias, and cerebrovascular accidents, has been explored in recent years. While different in many ways, including but not limited to symptom manifestations and etiologies, this group of conditions is essentially characterized by the effects of disease and/or injury on the delivery of blood supply to the brain and other organs, especially the ways in which deficiency in blood supply may affect motor strength, vision, balance, control and coordination as well as consciousness and cognition.

Heart Disease and Arrhythmias

It is not unreasonable to think that persons with cardiovascular problems would have higher crash rates, particularly patients with severe conditions. Consistent with such a notion, studies from Washington and California found nearly a two-fold increase in crash risk for drivers known to have heart disease (Waller, 1967; Crancer & O'Neall, 1970). However, Naughton et al. (1982) found that drivers hospitalized with ischemic heart disease did not show an increase in crashes over other drivers and failed to find an increase in accident rate for those with more severe disease.

Studying driving risks of patients after resuscitation from near-fatal ventricular tachyarrhythmia, Akiyama et al. (2001) compared patients on anti-arrhythmic drug therapies to others with implantable cardiac defibrillators using a questionnaire about driving habits and experiences. Interestingly, the group found that 57% of patients resumed driving within 3 months, 78% by 6 months, and 88% within 12 months; 2% had syncopal events while driving, 11% dizziness or palpitations that required stopping, and 8% defibrillator patients received shock. There were relatively few accidents (i.e., 3.4% during 1619 patient-years of follow-up). The authors concluded that most patients resume driving early after life-threatening tachyarrhythmia; additionally, it was common for patients to have symptoms but uncommon for them to be involved in accidents.

Other studies provided general support for the conclusion that, while large numbers of patients continued to driver after implantation, the incidence of accidents was relatively low in patients with implantable cardioverter defibrillators. Trappe et al. (1998) found that 59% of patients continued to drive post-implant with only rare occurrence of device-related syncopal events and no occurrences related to accidents. Results of a questionnaire by Finch et al. (1993) revealed that 70% of patients resumed driving within 8 months after implantation, half driving on a daily basis; 91% felt safe and comfortable while driving. Curtis et al. (1995) surveyed physicians about the safety in patients at risk for sudden death after device implantation; they found that about 10% of all defibrillators discharged during driving over 12 years with an estimated fatality rate and injury rate less than estimated injury rate for the general population. Interestingly, however, while concluding that there is a low risk of arrhythmic events behind-the-wheel, several studies suggested that concurrent medical problems imposed by driving may affect the ability of some drivers to deal with the more demanding driving tasks and increase risk by altering oxygenation or cardiac conduction (Bellet et al., 1968; Waller, 1992; Beauregard et al., 1995).

Stroke

While a comprehensive review of research related to stroke is presented in earlier chapters, it should be noted here that stroke is one of the most common cardiovascular-related disorders that can impact driving performance capacity. Individuals who suffer a cerebrovascular accident, or stroke, generally manifest more deficiencies in all measured areas of function and often experience physical, cognitive, and psychomotor dysfunction thought to be related to driving skills and abilities (Frier & Wilson, 1986). Most studies have focused on assessment of skills using off-road (e.g., pre-driver evaluations, simulators) and on-road methods and tests and identifying driving-related deficiencies (van Zomeren et al., 1987; Galski et al., 1990; Lings & Jensen, 1991; Galski et al., 1992, 1993; Heikkila et al., 1999; Klavora et al., 2000). While resulting in a compendium of abilities regarded as important in driving and finding that various methods of evaluation may be helpful in minimizing risks associated with on-road evaluation of potentially unsafe drivers, few studies have investigated the relationship of impairments, alone or in combination, to real-world accidents and/or crash risk.

OTHER MEDICAL CONDITIONS

The effect on driving of specific neurological disorders, including sleep disorders, seizures, multiple sclerosis (MS), age-related cognitive impairment and dementia, has been increasingly studied over the years. While some of these topics have been discussed in previous chapters, some additional considerations are presented.

Sleep Disorders

Sleepiness is regarded by many as a common cause of motor vehicle accidents with costs from damages in the range of billions of dollars each year. While it has been estimated that 2–3% of accidents are related to sleepiness, one study in Iceland suggested that over 15% of respondents to a questionnaire claimed sleepiness as a cause of single-car accidents (Gislason et al., 1997).

Recognizing the importance of controlled studies about the relationship between sleep disorders and driving, Masa et al. (2000) interviewed over 4,000 randomly selected drivers to look at driving performance, characteristics, and crash rates of sleepy drivers. They found that 3.6% of the sample could be characterized as habitually sleepy drivers who had several fold more accidents than controls; accidents were at least partially explained by respiratory disorders during sleep.

Other researchers also found that patients with a variety of sleep disorders had an increased risk of accidents. For example, Aldrich (1989) compared a group of healthy controls to patients with several kinds of sleep disorders, that is, apnea, narcolepsy, and other disorders with and without excessive sleepiness. Notably, hypersomnolent patients more than controls were 1.5 to 4 times more likely to be involved in accidents. Narcoleptics and apneics together accounted for 71% of all sleep-related accidents; narcoleptics demonstrated the highest proportion of accidents while apneics were involved in more accidents because of greater number. Findley et al. (1989) compared the performance of patients with and without severe sleep apnea in driving simulators. Patients with apnea hit a greater number of road obstacles and, generally, performed significantly worse than controls. In another study, Findley et al. (1992) demonstrated that patients with untreated obstructive sleep apnea performed more poorly than those with treated sleep apnea and had 2–3 times more accidents than other drivers; additionally, it was found that patients treated with nasal continuous positive airway pressure improved performance. Barbe et al. (1998), exploring the relationship between sleep apnea syndrome and car accidents, assessed vigilance and driving performance in a simulator. After controlling for sleepiness, anxiety and depression, the study revealed that patients had significantly greater odds of accidents than controls and were much more likely to have had more than one accident. No clinical or physiological markers used to define sleep apnea syndrome were able to discriminate patients at higher risk of accidents, however.

Seizure Disorders

A seizure is a sudden, involuntary change in behavior, muscle control, sensation, consciousness and/or mental state as a consequence of an abnormal electrical discharge in the brain. The type of seizure varies depending on the location of electrical hypersynchronization in the brain and the type of problem causing the seizure. In many instances, the cause of a seizure is idiopathic and unidentifiable. However, there are many identified causes of seizures that can be grouped into four main categories: neurological (e.g., congenital brain malformation, brain tumor, head trauma, cerebral degeneration), cardiovascular (e.g., stroke), psychological (e.g., pseudo-seizure) and others (e.g., inborn errors of metabolism, intracranial infection, withdrawal states, iatrogenic drug reactions) (Schacter, 1998).

Waller (1965) was one of the first researchers to report that crash risk in drivers with a seizure disorder appeared to be twice the risk of other drivers. Since that time, several other researchers found elevated crash risks for patients with seizure disorder, also. For example, Popkin and Waller (1988) found that patients known to licensing authorities had 1.4 times as many crashes per 100 drivers as general population; however, the type of seizure and degree of seizure control as well as the amount and nature of driving among patients was unknown. Hansotia and Broste (1991), in a population-based retrospective cohort study of more than 30,000 patients with and without epilepsy and diabetes mellitus, found slightly increased risks of traffic accidents and moving violations in epileptic and diabetic patients as compared to the unaffected group over a 4-year period. In a subsequent study of conditions marked by loss of consciousness, Hansotia (1993) identified factors that contributed to recurrence of seizures and affected driving safety. The author found that young males under 25-years old had the highest risk of accidents; partial complex seizure type, history of drug toxicity with anticonvulsants, alcohol abuse, poor compliance for medications, and a history of psychiatric illness increased the risk.

Multiple Sclerosis

Multiple Sclerosis (MS) is a neurological disorder, common among young adults, resulting from damage to the myelin sheath surrounding nerve fibers of the central nervous system (CNS). Interfering with messages between the brain and other parts of the body, damage to the myelin causes an array of symptoms, including but not limited to fatigue, tingling, numbness, painful sensations, blurred or double vision, muscle weakness, impaired balance, spasticity, tremor, speech and dysphagia, and mood swings. According to the National Multiple Sclerosis Society Anonymous (2001), hearing loss occurs in about 6% of patients with MS, especially during periods of exacerbation, or flare-ups. Additionally, about 50% of people with MS develop some cognitive dysfunction, such as slowness in thinking, difficulty with memory, and problems in attention, concentration and reasoning; notably, only 10% of the group with cognitive dysfunction develop problems that are severe enough to interfere in a significant way with everyday activities.

Schultheis et al. (2001) studied the influence of cognitive impairment on driving performance in MS. The authors compared 13 MS patients with evidence of cognitive impairment on neuropsychological tests to 15 MS patients without signs of deficits in cognition and 17 healthy controls of similar age and driving experience on off-road measures of driving. In the absence of significant physical limitations, MS patients with cognitive impairments performed significantly worse than those without deficits and controls in response times to simulated driving scenarios and had a higher percentage regarded as a high risk of probable crash involvement.

Parkinson's Disease

Parkinson's disease (PD) is a chronic, progressive disorder of the CNS whose essential feature is degeneration of dopamine neurons of the substantia nigra and an abnormally low concentration of dopamine in the basal ganglia; it is a motor system disorder that primarily affects muscle movement and leads to characteristic symptoms, including tremors or shaking, stiffness or rigidity of the limbs and trunk, slowness of movement, difficulty in walking and talking, problems with balance and loss of coordination. Additionally, many patients manifest problems in cognition, for example, slowness in thinking and information processing and, notably, patients with PD have an almost six-fold increase in risk for dementia in comparison to those without the disorder (Aarsland et al., 2001). More than a million people in the United States currently live with PD and nearly 50,000 Americans every year are diagnosed with the disease. In about 5–10% of cases, PD begins before age 50; however, the first symptoms develop after age 50 for most people, and the likelihood of developing PD continues to increase with age.

In one study Dubinsky et al. (1991) found on the basis of interviews that patients with PD, overall, had no more lifetime accidents than controls. However, the authors found that there were more reported accidents in patients with severe PD and, as disability worsened over time, the smaller percentage of patients who continued to drive traveled fewer miles and experienced proportionately more accidents. Notably, cognitive impairment was associated with an increase in accident rate. Heikkila et al. (1998), in a study comparing 20 patients with idiopathic PD and 20 matched healthy controls in laboratory tests of cognition and psychomotor performance as well as a controlled driving test, concluded that driving ability was significantly decreased in patients with even mild to moderate PD. In other studies on the relationship between driving and PD, drivers with PD were often found to be impaired by characteristic motor symptoms but, additionally, by psychiatric complications, multi-morbidity, increased daytime sleepiness exacerbated by the sedative effects of dopiminergic agents used for treatment, and cognitive disturbances (Borromei et al., 1999; Lachenmayer, 2000).

Age-Related Cognitive Impairment and Dementia

The number of people who are 65 years of age or older in the United States is growing more rapidly than any other age group. By the year 2020, 17% of the population is expected to fall in this age range; estimates reach up to 50 million elderly who will be licensed or driving (Carr, 1993; Retchin & Anapolle, 1983).

Healthy aging brings remarkable changes in cardiorespiratory endurance, muscle strength, vision and hearing, neurologic function, immune response, and other areas of physiology (Moeller, 1989). Chronic medical illness increases in prevalence with advancing age; more than 80% of those older than 65 years of age have at least one chronic disease and the majority of this group have two or more.

While elderly drivers account for a lower proportion of accidents and crashes than any other age group, they have an increased risk on a per-mile basis for involvement in motor vehicle crashes (Graca, 1986). Older age has been linked to a higher risk of involvement in motor vehicle accidents consequent to changes in sensory (e.g., vision, hearing), motor and cognitive functions as well as medical conditions (e.g., cardiovascular disorders) and use of medications that can affect driving performance (Waller & Goo, 1969; Owsley et al., 1991; Retchin & Anapolle, 1983; Koepsell et al., 1994; Abrams et al., 1995; Fitten et al., 1995; Hemmelgarn et al., 1997; Sims et al., 1998; Gallo et al., 1999; Owsley et al., 1999). In addition to greater involvement in crashes, elderly drivers are more likely to die or suffer more serious injury in crashes; moreover, the elderly driver who survives a crash takes longer to recover in the hospital and is more likely to succumb to later secondary complications (Partyka, 1983; OECD, 1985; Waller, 1985; Evans, 1988; Reuben et al., 1988; Ball & Owsley, 1991; McGwin et al., 2000).

Complicating the relationship between age-related medical conditions and driving is dementia, a syndrome characterized by impairments in memory, judgment, abstract thought and other disturbances of higher cortical function and manifested in about 15% of persons over 65-years old (American Psychiatric Association, 1999). Based on neuropathologic studies, Alzheimer's disease (AD), the most common cause, accounts for dementia in 50–70% of older patients and multiple infarct dementia in an additional 15–25% of patients (Mortimer, 1983; Terry & Katzman, 1983).

Waller (1967) was one of the first researchers to compare the frequency of accidents and traffic violations in normal and older drivers with dementia and cardiovascular disease. Interestingly, after adjusting for number of driven miles, the accident rate was almost twice as high for those with dementia and 4 times as high among those with combined dementia and cardiovascular disease. Traffic violations were statistically higher only for patients with dementia and cardiovascular disease in comparison to normal elderly drivers.

Others have found an increase in crashes for persons with dementia, also. Comparing 30 probable AD patients and 20 matched control subjects with similar amounts of driving, Friedland et al. (1988) found that 47% of patients had at least one accident compared to 10% for the controls; there was nearly an eight-fold greater risk of an accident in the 31–35% who continued to drive after diagnosis in comparison to controls. Interestingly, most crashes involved errors at intersections and occurred at early and middle stages of the disease; the authors concluded that dementia severity and duration were not directly related to crashes. In a later meta-analytic study of crash rates for patients with Alzheimer's dementia, Carr (1997) found that 50% stopped driving within 3 years of diagnosis; males were at increased risk. The risk for crashes increased with duration of driving after onset. Dementia severity did not correlate with risk for crash; additional medical conditions were regarded as a factor in crash risk.

In a driving survey of relatives and caregivers, Lucas-Blaustein et al. (1988) compared a small sample of current and discontinued drivers with dementia of the Alzheimer's type, multi-infarct dementia and other types of unknown etiology. They found that 30% were involved in crashes and 11% caused crashes. Drachman and Swearer (1993) used a questionnaire to determine risk of crashes among 130 AD patients who continued to drive after onset compared to 112 age-matched normal subjects. The AD patients were found to have had more crashes per year in comparison to controls but only a moderately greater rate in comparison to drivers of all ages. A closer look at the findings revealed that the average number of crashes changed each year of driving after onset of dementia; the moderate crash rates reflected reduction in exposure with longer drivers experiencing significantly more crashes.

Trobe et al. (1996) investigated car crash and violation rates for 143 AD patients and 715 licensed elderly comparison subjects. Crash and violation rates for AD patients were not significantly different from comparisons; the authors concluded that findings did not confirm an reportedly excessive crash rate among drivers with AD relative to an appropriate comparison group. Rizzo et al. (1997), in an effort to measure relevant performance using a high fidelity simulator, examined effect of AD on collision avoidance in a small sample of patients and controls. The authors found that 29% of AD patients had crashes in comparison to none of the controls but, notably, AD patients were more than twice as likely to experience close calls. Visuospatial impairment, reduction in useful field of view, reduced perception of dimensional structures from motion predicted crashes. In another study, Rizzo et al. (2001) found similar rates for crashes in comparable demented and non-demented groups. Based on analysis of collision avoidance in a simulator, the authors suggested that crashes in cognitively impaired older drivers were related to failure to notice other drivers at intersections.

DIABETES MELLITUS

According to the American Medical Association (1986), about one-third of diabetics have insulin-dependent (Type 1) diabetes and approximately two-thirds, including most diabetics 65 and older, have non-insulin-dependent (Type 2) diabetes. Hypoglycemic unawareness, characterized by a decrease in alertness and disorientation without a person's recognition, is a recognized complication of Type I and Type 2 diabetes. Sometimes extreme hypoglycemia can result in altered consciousness, coma or convulsions. The sudden occurrence of disabling hypoglycemia and the long-term consequences of the disease, especially changes in vision (e.g., retinopathy), have been thought to make drivers more prone to accidents than the average driver. Additionally, there is a concern that efforts by physicians in recent years to improve glycemic control of diabetes and avoid the late stage renal, cardiac, and visual complications frequently associated with the disease by intensive glucose-lowering agents and tighter regimens on a daily basis may actually induce episodes of hypoglycemia-related alterations in consciousness that can affect driving (DCCT Research Group, 1987; Ehrlich, 1991).

Much of the available research has shown that the crash experiences of diabetic drivers are greater in comparison to other drivers (Waller, 1965; Frier et al., 1980; Laberge-Nadeau et al., 2000). One study found that diabetic drivers in America had nearly double the accident rate of other drivers (Crancer & McMurray, 1968). Another study revealed a modest increase in crash risk for a sample of diabetics; notably, however, there was no distinction between insulin and non-insulin users in the study (Hansotia & Broste, 1991). Veneman (1996), using computer simulation techniques, showed that moderate hypoglycemia significantly worsened driving performance and caused motor vehicle accidents. Interestingly, the author found decreased incidence of hypoglycemia and demonstrated less involvement of diabetics in crashes (crash rates 6.8 versus 29.8 per 1,000,000 miles) after discovering that unawareness of accident-related changes in blood glucose was a major risk factor in accident-related errors and adapting a special glucose awareness training program that facilitated early detection of changes in glucose levels.

Cox et al. (1993), considering the notion that diabetic hypoglycemia produces cognitive-motor slowing that can increase risk of crashes, manipulated blood glucose levels during performance in a driving simulator. Performance was not disrupted at a mildly hypoglycemic level or even after recovery from moderately low levels. However, moderate hypoglycemia adversely affected patients' steering ability and caused more swerving, spinning, time over road midline and time off the road; moreover, it resulted in compensatory slowing down while driving. These driving decrements were observed in 35% of patients and were reportedly unrelated to demographic, disease or unfavorable driving histories. In a more recent study, Cox et al. (2000) evaluated the blood glucose level at which driving became impaired as well as patients' detection of impairment and corrective action. Results indicated that, while driving performance was significantly disrupted with relatively mild hypoglycemia, patients demonstrated hesitation to take any corrective action until experiencing an increase in neurological symptoms; the researchers concluded that delay in treatment produced neuroglycopenia, which precluded corrective behaviors and placed drivers at increased risk for motor vehicle accidents. In another study, Cox et al. (2001) further demonstrated that driving was affected by cognitive impairment resulting from episodes of hypoglycemia and noted that intensive insulin therapy can increase the likelihood of severe hypoglycemia. The group also found in simulator tests that driving had an intrinsic metabolic demand which contributed to hypoglycemia and ultimately to accidents while driving with low blood glucose.

Some researchers have suggested that older individuals are at greater risk of accidents because hypoglycemic episodes increase with age while the adrenergic response alerting the patient of a hypoglycemic episode decreases with age (Jennings et al., 1989). However, in one study which examined the association between diabetes, its complications and at-fault automobile crashes among older drivers, no association between diabetes and at-fault crash involvement. The study provided no evidence that older drivers with diabetes are at increased risk for automobile crashes (McGwin et al., 2000).

On the other hand, several researchers have not found any significant increase in crash risk for diabetic drivers as a group. For example, Songer et al. (1988) found no appreciable increase in crash risk although, interestingly, noted gender differences, that is, higher risk for women than men. Eadington and Frier (1989), who reviewed the self-reported driving habits and experiences of Type I diabetics and a matched group of respondents to a questionnaire, concluded that the accident rate was relatively infrequent and comparable to the rate of accidents for the non-diabetic driving population of similar age. The rate of accidents was higher for females (6.3 per million miles) than for males (4.9 per million miles).

PSYCHIATRIC MORBIDITY

Patients with mental illness, such as depression and schizophrenia, may be regarded as more liable to accidents than others because of associated impairments in attention and concentration, anxiety, agitation or retardation, riskiness or carelessness, fatigue, substance abuse, and side effects of medications used for treatment.

Some studies suggested that schizophrenic patients violate traffic regulations more often than non-psychiatric population but other studies have found no differences between the groups. Edlund et al. (1989) compared 103 out-patient schizophrenic patients and an age-matched sample of 123 controls. Significantly fewer schizophrenic patients drove in comparison to controls; those who drove traveled fewer miles but had more accidents per miles driven. The authors concluded that there was a greater risk of motor vehicle accidents per miles driven in schizophrenics who chose to drive. In Israel, Schlosberg (1990) found no increase in traffic violations and fines for a sample of 82 schizophrenics in comparison to a control group or any difference between paranoid and non-paranoid patients.

In a Swiss study, Niveau and Kelley-Puskas (2001) compared driving records of psychiatric patients reported to medical authorities to determine if they represented a higher risk of accidents and traffic violations than unreported drivers. The authors were unable to conclude that there were any significant differences between psychiatric patients and normal in accidents and violations in light of evidence that reporting was not objective.

Kazniak et al. (1991) compared 21 patients with mild dementia due to AD to 18 patients with major depression and memory difficulties matched for age, education, and sex. A significantly larger number of depressed patients continued to drive than patients with dementia (72% and 14%, respectively) but those with dementia had a slightly higher accident rate than depressives (29% and 11%, respectively).

MEDICATIONS

Medications, alone or in combination, are used by people of all ages to treat a variety of acute and chronic medical conditions; amelioration of suffering, restoration of physical condition and health, and cure from disease are produced by the effects of medications on physiological functions. However, many medications used to treat disorders and diseases can adversely interfere with physiological functioning, particularly CNS functioning, or exacerbate the effects of medical conditions on driving in indeterminable ways.

Experimental and epidemiological studies of adults showed that some medications impair driving performance and elevate risk of crashes (Seppala et al., 1979; Cowart & Kandela, 1985; Linnoila et al., 1986; Polen & Friedman, 1988; McGwin et al., 2000). And, as the number of persons 65 years of age and older increases in America, there has been a growing concern about the effects of medications on driving performance in this group.

Notably, medication use increases with age and is common in those 65 years of age and older; this age group, which comprises approximately 12% of the population in the United States, receives about 32% of dispensed prescription drugs and fills an average of nearly 20 prescriptions each year (HCFA, 1988). And, perhaps because older individuals are more susceptible to the adverse CNS effects resulting from age-related pharmacodynamic changes or decline in hepatic and renal function required for the elimination of many medications, there is a high frequency and severity of adverse side effects in the elderly (Ray et al., 1992; Ray et al., 1993). Adding to the concern is the concurrent use of multiple medications with resultant additive or synergistic interactions can produce adverse CNS effects (Salzman, 1985). It is common in the elderly and frequently the cause of hospitalization for delirium (Kurfees & Dotson, 1987; Francis et al., 1990; Kroenke & Pinholt, 1990). One study indicated than 80% of those 65 and older receive one or more prescribed medication (e.g., benzodiazepines, cyclic antidepressant, antipsychotics, antihistamines, narcotic analgesics, and hypoglycemics) (Moeller & Mathiowetz, 1989).

BENZODIAZEPINES

Benzodiazepines are the most frequently prescribed medications for the treatment of anxiety and insomnia (Ray et al., 1992). Basically, there are two groups of benzodiazepines: (1) the long-acting drugs, such as diazepam (e.g., Valium), chlordiazepoxide (e.g., Librium), clorazepate (e.g., Tranxene), and flurazepam (e.g., Dalmane), which have half-life of at least 24 hours and require complex hepatic biotransformation before elimination, and (2) the short-acting drugs, including alprazolam (e.g., Xanax), oxazepam (e.g., Serax), lorazepam (e.g., Ativan), triazolam (e.g., Halcion), and temazepam (e.g., Restoril), which have elimination half-life of less than 24 hours and are biotransformed through less complex metabolic pathways. The effects of benzodiazepines on the CNS include drowsiness, confusion, ataxia, dizziness, decreased motor coordination, and impaired memory and recall.

Although often effective in promoting tranquility and sleep, it has been suggested that benzodiazepines lead to substantial impairment in psychomotor functioning and an increased risk of motor vehicle accidents (Barbone et al., 1998; McGwin et al, 2000). In support of this conclusion, studies using controlled driving tests or measurements of driving-related skills (e.g., choice reaction time, divided attention, visual stimulus detection, hand–eye coordination) have consistently found that benzodiazepines impaired performance shortly after ingestion (Palva et al., 1982; Hindmarch 1986; Seppala et al., 1986). For some drug–dose combinations, Mortimer and Howat (1986) found impairment almost equivalent to the effect produced by moderate (0.10%) blood alcohol levels. Anther study using open-road evaluations have examined the effects of medication on driving ability by measuring the standard deviation of a vehicle's lateral position (SDLP), or vehicular weaving (Menzin et al., 2000). Findings indicated that a relatively slight change of 2.5cm in SDLP, which is equivalent to 0.05% Blood Alcohol Concentration (BAC), resulted in a 25% increased risk of a motor vehicle accident by weaving (Menzin et al., 2000). Skegg et al. (1979), in a prospective study of over 43,000 people prescribed medications by general practitioners, found a highly significant association between the use of minor tranquilizers and an almost five-fold increase in risk of a serious road accident. Thomas (1998), examining the relationship between benzodiazepine use and accidents in case-control studies, found that medication use almost doubles the risk of motor vehicle accidents.

Age-related decreases in the efficiency of metabolic pathways utilized by these medications extend their half-lives in older patients and increase sensitivity to their effects as well as the duration and intensity of side effects (Reidenberg et al.,

1978; Regestein, 1984; Salzman, 1984). Studies have found that traffic accident risk increases by nearly 50% in the first week after starting benzodiazepine therapy (Hemmelgarn et al., 1997). Brief or extended periods of exposure to long half-life benzodiazepines have been found to produce a hypnotic, or "hang over" effect the next day that impaired cognition and motor behaviors and was linked to crash involvement where at least one person sustained bodily injury (O'Hanlon & Volkerts, 1986; Hemmelgarn et al., 1997).

Additionally, others have argued that benzodiazepines adversely affect the safety of the older driver, particularly for high doses and long half-life compounds (Reidel et al., 1988; Thomas, 1998; Ray et al., 1993). In one study, O'Hanlon and Volkerts (1986) examined the effects of two long-acting hypnotics, that is, nitrazepam (e.g., Mogadon) and temazepam, on actual driving in primary highway circuit and normal traffic. Results indicated that nitrazepam adversely affected driving performance throughout the active medication period; however, temazepam produced no adverse effects. Another study found little adverse effects on higher mental functioning with diazepam and chlordiazepoxide; however, it was suggested that these medications slow down simple repetitive motor actions similar to those seemingly required in driving (Murray, 1984).

ANTIHISTAMINES

Antihistamines are commonly prescribed to alleviate allergy symptoms and may also be used as hypnotics. These medications are classified as first-generation (diphenhydramine [e.g., Benadryl], doxylamine [e.g., Unisom]) or second-generation (e.g., loratadine [Claritin], fexofenadine [e.g., Allegra], cetirizine [e.g., Zyrtec], terfenadine [e.g., Seldane]) antihistamines. First-generation antihistamines readily cross the blood brain barrier and result in sedating effects on the CNS which include drowsiness, altered mood, reduced wakefulness, impaired cognitive performance, and psychomotor coordination (Kay & Harris, 1999). Sedating antihistamines are also associated with compromised performance in psychomotor tasks that require a high degree of alertness or concentration (Philpot, 2000; Settipane, 1999). According to Meltzer (1990), sedation occurs in 10–25% of antihistamine users. Second-generation (H1-receptor antagonist) antihistamines do not cross the blood brain barrier and thus are largely free from the CNS effects of sedating antihistamines (Gengo et al., 1989).

Despite the sedation associated with first-class antihistamines (e.g., diphenhydramine), some physicians continue to prescribe these older medications for allergy sufferers and patients continue to use drugs in this class that may not require medical consultation, prescription or monitoring. Sedating antihistamines are often found to be a causal factor in fatal traffic accidents and, interestingly, are the leading medication found on autopsy of pilots who have crashed their aircraft (Kay & Quig, 2001).

Kay and Harris (1999) found that first-class antihistamines had significant adverse effects on driving-related abilities, such as vigilance, divided attention, working memory, and psychomotor performance. O'Hanlon and Ramaekers (1995) studied effects of antihistamines on driving performance, specifically, impairment in vehicular weaving between lanes (i.e., SDLP). Impairment in driving performance was found with sedating antihistamines and associated with dosage, time after ingestion, and repeated doses after 4–5 days. Others have found that many who use these antihistamines manifest deficits in cognitive and psychomotor functioning prior to awareness of the medication's sedating effects; consequently, drivers experienced difficulties in following distances, lane control, and steering stability without realization of operating problems (Gengo & Manning, 1990; Kay & Harris, 1999; Bloomfield et al., 2000).

The most commonly prescribed second-generation antihistamines include loratadine, fexofenadine, and cetirizine. Several studies have found that loratadine and cetirizine at their therapeutic levels did not produce sedation or impair cognitive-motor performance (Gengo & Manning, 1990; Hansen, 1999; Kay & Harris, 1999; Philpot, 2000). Similarly, fexofenadine did not impair driving performance when assessed for driving safety; on the contrary, driving performance was consistently better with fixed dosages per day of fexofenadine than placebo (Vermeeren & O'Hanlon, 1998). Additionally, two older antihistamines in this class (i.e., terfenadine and astemizole [e.g., Hismanal]) given at therapeutic levels in single and multiple doses were never found to impair driving performance and other psychomotor skills; notably, however, these medications are no longer available by prescription (Aaronson, 1993).

ANTICONVULSANTS

Anticonvulsant medications used to treat epilepsy and other seizure disorders are directed at restoring neuronal function to normal; some are also used in the treatment of affective disorders, such as bipolar illness, and chronic pain syndromes, such as trigeminal neuralgia. Phenobarbital and phenytoin (e.g., Dilantin) are among the oldest anticonvulsants still in use for epilepsy; carbamazepine (e.g., Tegretol) and divalproex sodium (e.g., Depakote) have been used widely for treating epilepsy as well as depression and pain. More recently, second-generation antiepileptic drugs (felbamate [e.g., Felbatol], gabapentin [e.g., Neurotin], lamotrigine [e.g., Lamictal], topiramate [e.g., Topimax], tiagabine [e.g., Gabitril]) have become available. Depending on the medication and dosage, neurotoxic side effects of anticonvulsants include drowsiness and somnolence, dizziness, ataxia, blurred or double vision, cognitive changes, and confusion (Albers et al., 2001).

Research has been limited on the effects of anticonvulsant medications on driving and studies have shown varying results depending on populations and selected outcome measures (Novak, 1991). However, Hansotia (1993a, b) found that drivers with episodic disorders may have up to twice the risk of crashes and moving violations compared to the general population or age-matched controls. Others have suggested an increased risk for motor vehicle crashes associated with loss of consciousness in epilepsy and seizure disorders (Barolin & Haslinger, 1991; Fukushima, 1991; Laubichler, 1992). Hasegawa et al. (1991), who surveyed 72 drivers with epilepsy, found that 25% reported at least one crash due to seizure and 10% of the crashes, mostly minor, were caused by partial seizures. Hashimoto (1991) reported that 9% of 81 drivers with epilepsy had crashes over a 5-year period but none due to seizures.

ANTIDEPRESSANTS

Antidepressants can be placed into several main categories based on distinct pharmacologic mechanisms. The two time-honored mechanisms are the tricyclic antidepressants (TCAs: amitriptyline [e.g., Elavil], clomipramine [e.g., Anafranil], nortriptyline [e.g., Pamelor], doxepin [e.g., Sinequan], imipramine [e.g., Tofranil]) and the monoamine oxidase inhibitors (MAOIs: isocarboxazid [e.g., Marplan], tranylcypromine [e.g., Parnate], phenelzine [e.g., Nardil); the more recent and most widely prescribed agents are the selective serotonin reuptake inhibitors (SSRIs: citalopram [e.g., Celexa], fluoxetine [e.g., Prozac], fluvoxamine [e.g., Luvox], paroxetine [e.g., Paxil], sertraline [e.g., Zoloft]). There are several other classes which, like the SSRIs, increase serotonergic transmission but, additionally, have other actions (mirtazapine [e.g., Remeron], nefazodone [e.g., Serzone], trazodone [e.g., Desyrel]); and, there is a novel class in which the selective norepinephrine and dopamine reuptake inhibitor has no direct actions on the serotonin system (buproprion [e.g., Wellbutrin]) (Stahl, 1998). Additionally, medications called mood stabilizers (e.g., lithium, carbamazepine) are often used with antidepressants to facilitate recovery from affective disorders, particularly bipolar disorders.

Adverse reactions to antidepressants and mood stabilizers vary depending mostly on the class of medication and dosage. However, susceptibility to side effects may be related to age, also. Generally, side effects of antidepressants include sedation and somnolence, postural hypotension, dizziness, blurred or double vision, psychomotor retardation, and cognitive changes.

Harvey (1985) argued that cyclic antidepressants have sedative effects which impair psychomotor functioning. In another study, Hindmarch and Subhan (1986) found that the TCAs, amitriptyline and trazodone, have a detrimental effect on cognitive, psychomotor and driving ability. Van Laar et al. (1995) found that nefazodone and imipramine were associated with sedation and daytime sleepiness. Similar results were found by Robbe and O'Hanlon (1995) for actual driving and psychomotor performance with paroxetine.

Researchers have argued that the newer class of antidepressants, SSRIs, tend to show less behavioral toxicity (Soyka et al., 1998). Reportedly, SSRIs result in fewer side effects and, therefore, may not impair driving ability (Hindmarch & Easton, 1990). However, recent laboratory studies that have investigated the effects of antidepressants on driving performance, have not supported this conclusion unequivocally. For example, O'Hanlon et al. (1998), investigating the effects of venlafaxine (Effexor) on off-road and on-road measures regarded as important in driving, found significant impairment in driving-related vigilance. The authors suggested that interference with 5-HT transmission reduced arousal, particularly in monotonous tasks or environments. Similarly, when Hatcher et al. (1990) examined the effects of a mood stabilizer (e.g., Lithium) on driving by using a computerized driving simulator, results indicated reduced reaction time and tracking ability along with an increase in driving errors.

ANTIPSYCHOTICS

Neuroleptics, or major tranquilizers, are used primarily for the treatment of schizophrenia and other psychotic disorders, which are often marked by disturbed or bizarre thinking (e.g., hallucinations, delusions), and for control of agitated behavior associated with organic disorders, such as dementia (Spira et al., 1984). Antipsychotics can be distinguished by their pharmacology, action at receptors and clinical properties. Typical antipsychotics (e.g., haloperidol [e.g., Haldol], thioridazine [e.g., Mellaril], chlorpromazine [e.g., Thorazine], thiothixene [e.g., Navane], and trifluoperazine [e.g., Stelazine]) act primarily at dopamine receptors. Atypical antipsychotics (clozapine [e.g., Clorazil], risperidone [e.g., Risperdal], olanzapine [e.g., Zyprexa]) affect other neurotransmitter systems, including serotonin, or have selective affinity for specific dopamine receptors (Abrams et al., 1995). Antipsychotics, which are structurally similar to cyclic antidepressants, can produce a wide range of side effects. Sedation, fatigue, and weakness are common side effects of neuroleptic treatment as well as anticholinergic effects marked by light-headedness, dizziness and blurred vision. Additionally, these medications, especially the typical antipsychotics, can result in extrapyramidal side effects, including Parkinson-like symptoms (e.g., rigidity, tremor, bradykinesia, and dystonia) and tardive dyskinesia marked by purposeless movements. Some increase the risk of convulsions.

Despite the widespread use of antipsychotics, Judd (1985), noting that tolerance to sedation and decreased alertness occurs with regular treatment, found little evidence that these medications were significantly implicated in vehicular crashes or deaths. Other studies, however, found that neuroleptic use was associated with impaired performance in off-road tests and measures of driving-related abilities. For example, Wylie et al. (1993) compared 22 chronic schizophrenic patients receiving depot neuroleptics (i.e., slow release forms of typical antipsychotics) to 16 control subjects in their performance on simulated driving tests. The authors found a significant decrement in driving performance for the index group compared to normal controls. Grabe et al. (1999), studying the effects of neuroleptic medication and co-medication in regard to driving fitness, compared a small sample of patients receiving clozapine to others using classical neuroleptics. Both treatment groups were equally impaired on measures of reaction time, vigilance, visual perception, and stress tolerance.

ANTI-PARKINSONIANS

Because there is no known cure for PD, treatment is aimed at controlling the symptoms with medications, especially medications that increase supply of dopamine to improve movement and balance (levodopa/carbodopa [e.g., Sinemet], deprenyl [e.g., Seligene], bromocriptine [e.g., Parlodel], pergolide [e.g., Permax], pramipexole [e.g., Mirapex], ropinirole [e.g., Requip]). Additionally, other medications, such as antidepressants and antihistamines, are commonly used in the treatment of PD to control side effects of the primary medications.

Many of the anti-parkinsonian medications can cause severe side effects, including systemic disorders, involuntary movements, depression, confusion, delusions, agitation, paranoid ideation, and cognitive deficits. And, the adjunctive medications concomitantly used in treatment have been linked to memory loss, blurred vision, changes in mental activity, and confusion.

Moreover, because of the pathology of PD and the dopaminergic drugs used in treatment, patients can experience a number of sleep disorders, including insomnia, parasomnias and daytime somnolence, such as excessive daytime sleepiness (EDS) and "sleep attacks" (Moller et al., 2000). Excessive daytime sleepiness is, in fact, common in PD patients (Hauser et al., 2000; Larsen & Tandberg, 2001). However, it has not been found to be unique to one medication over the other; researchers have consistently found that all dopamine agonists used to treat PD are associated with increased sedation and EDS. And, notably, EDS related to use of these medications worsens with increased age, advanced disease, and increased treatment dose (Lachenmayer, 2000; Pals et al., 2001).

Lings and Dupont (1992) compared the driving performance in a mock car of 28 persons suffering from PD and 109 healthy controls. They found that the PD patients with presumed optimal drug regimens and without complicating disorders, failed in reacting to stimuli on several occasions, demonstrated a high frequency of erroneous reactions in particular directional errors, and manifested reduced strength, speed of movement and increased reaction times characterized by prolongation of the reaction distance when driving a car at a higher speed.

Several recent studies have examined the occurrence of sudden "sleep attacks" in PD patients and, generally, found an increased risk of impairment in driving ability with the use of dopamine agonist medications (Frucht et al., 1999; Lachenmayer, 2000; Miranda et al., 2001; Moller, 2001). Ondo et al. (2001), noting that dopamine agonists had been causally implicated in motor vehicle accidents, studied the effects of the three most common dopamine agonists (i.e., pramipexole, ropinirole, pergolide) on daytime sleepiness in 320 Parkinson's patients over a 3-month period. Results indicated that the soporific effects of the medications were similar. Additionally, the authors found that falling asleep while driving was reported by almost 23% of current drivers and correlated significantly with higher scores on a measure of sleepiness.

NARCOTIC ANALGESICS

Advances in medicine have resulted in a wide variety of treatments and medications for acute and chronic non-malignant and malignant pain. Common treatments include non-aspirin pain relievers (e.g., acetaminophen), anti-inflammatory drugs (e.g., aspirin), steroidal drugs (e.g., cortisol, prednisone), and non-steroidal anti-inflammatories (NSAIDs: e.g., ibuprofen). Generally, these medications do not produce side effects that interfere with driving ability. Morphine-like drugs, called opioids (e.g., codeine, hydromorphone [e.g., Dilaudid], propoxyphene [e.g., Darvon], oxycodone [e.g., OxyContin], meperidine [e.g., Demerol], methadone), are prescribed for the treatment of moderate to severe acute pain and cancer pain and occasionally for certain chronic, non-cancer pain, also. Side effects from opioids are prevalent; the most common side effects include constipation, nausea, vomiting, and some degree of sedation.

In studies of single dose opioid treatment, studies have shown inconsistent findings in effects on driving ability. For example, Sjogren et al. (1994) found that single dose opioid treatment did not impair psychomotor functioning while Vainio et al. (1995) found that single dose opioid therapy administered to healthy volunteers impaired reaction time, muscle coordination, attention, and short-term memory sufficiently enough to affect driving.

Additionally, little is known about the effects of long-term opioid therapy on real-world driving despite increasing use of oral opioids and other narcotic analgesics in the treatment of cancer and non-malignant pain syndromes (Larsen et al., 1999). Several studies have determined that long-term opioid use has little or only mild and selective effects on psychomotor and cognitive abilities regarded as important in driving (Vainio et al., 1995; Zacny, 1995). Epidemiological studies have provided general support for the conclusions that opioid users do not experience more accidents or driving violations than non-users and that risk tended to vary with the type of drug (Babst et al., 1973; Blomberg & Preusser, 1974; Gordon, 1976; Budd et al., 1989; Ray et al., 1992; Galski et al., 2000; Meijler, 2000).

On the other hand, some researchers have found that these analgesics interfere with psychomotor function, muscle coordination, reaction time, and cognitive abilities required in driving performance. Additionally, epidemiological studies have linked to a higher risk of motor vehicle accidents resulting in injuries, driving violations, and infractions when these drugs are used for the long-term treatment of pain (Blomberg & Preusser, 1974; Gordon, 1976; Budd et al., 1989; Kerr et al., 1991; Ray et al., 1992; Sjogren et al., 1994; Vainio et al., 1995; Meijler, 2000).

Others have found that effects on driving performance may depend on the specific medication in use. For example, Starmer (1986), in reviewing the effects of analgesics on driving performance, found that codeine, meperidine and methadone impaired motor skills on a simulated driving task; however, similar effects were not found for propoxyphene.

CARDIOVASCULAR MEDICATIONS

Cardiovascular medications are used for the treatment of hypertension, abnormal heart rhythms, coronary artery disease, angina and other cardiac and circulatory problems. Commonly used medications for cardiovascular conditions include Beta adrenergic blocking agents (atenolol [e.g., Tenormin], metoprolol [e.g., Lopressor], propranolol [Inderal], sotolol [e.g., Betapace]) and angiotensin-converting enzyme inhibitors ([e.g., benzaperil [e.g., Lotensin], quinapril [e.g., accupril], enalapril [e.g., Vasotec]). Driving-related side effects include sleepiness, light-headedness and dizziness, especially with agents (e.g., propranolol, metoprolol) that easily pass the blood/brain barrier and enter the CNS in high concentrations.

The research on the effects of cardiovascular medication, namely beta blocking antihypertensive agents, on driving ability is limited, however. One study by Betts (1981) suggested that the sedating effects of specific medications in this class may lead to driving impairments marked by a decrease in visual acuity, alertness and reaction ability. Other studies have not revealed any contraindications for driving while using antihypertensive medications and, in fact, have consistently found no impairment in driving abilities in patients using antihypertensive medications, particularly the class of antihypertensives (e.g., atenolol) that do not readily cross the blood/brain barrier (John, 1980; Willumeit et al., 1984; McGwin et al., 2000). Still other studies have found improved visual acuity, decreased diastolic and systolic blood pressures and, in some cases, improved driving ability with an associated decrease in subjective stress while using the antihypertensive, atenolol (Clayton et al., 1977; Dunn et al., 1979; Panizza & Lecasble, 1985).

SUMMARY AND CONCLUSIONS

The current review of the literature was undertaken in an effort to (a) collect studies which have demonstrated the effects of medical conditions and medications on a person's ability to safely operate a motor vehicle as measured by real-world outcomes, including accidents, crashes and traffic violations and (b) determine from available research, if possible, the extent to which driving is compromised by illness and medications. The following conclusions came out of this review:

• While only a sample has been collected in this review, the large number of studies conducted in this country along with evidence of increased research interests in other countries over the past several decades reflected the expanding recognition that traffic safety is inextricably linked to human frailty and illness as well as to the treatments brought to bear on improving or ameliorating these conditions.

• When evaluated in terms of the selected outcome criteria, that is, accidents traffic violations, many medical conditions and medications apparently result in elevated risks. However, the medical diagnoses and medications per se did not predict the extent of risk (Mola, 1995).

• Medical conditions and medications compromise driving safety by their effects on functional ability, that is, the integration of physical and cognitive abilities, rather than by deficits in anatomy and physiology associated with a disease (Retchin, 1989; Wallace & Retchin, 1992).

• Inconsistencies, sometimes contradictions in findings about the relationship between driving, medical conditions and medications are evident between and within medical populations and stand out as a major problem affecting validity of conclusions, generalization of results and, ultimately, decisions about fitness to drive. A number of methodological issues are at the center of this problem: diagnostic inaccuracy; difficulty in defining people with the alleged condition due to limitations of current procedures for classification; problems in determining severity of illness; contamination of the studied population by co-morbidities and mixes of conditions; problems in partialing out the effects of treatment on the medical condition under study and/or co-morbid conditions; trouble in carrying out cohort studies with small samples of drivers who have the medical condition or use the medication under study; frequent lack of information about medications, including type, dosages, intervals and between doses; and, the complexities involved in studying the effects of multiple diseases and multiple medications with multiple doses (Waller, 1992).

• Revealed in the numerous surveys, questionnaires, off-road and on-road tests in cited studies, the absence of any standardized methods for assessing driving performance opens interpretation and comparison of results to discussion.

REFERENCES

Aaronson, D. W. (1993). Effects of terfenadine on psychomotor performance. An overview. *Drug Saf.*, *8*(4), 321–329.

Aarsland, D., Anderson, K., Larsen, J. P., Lolk, A., Nielsen, H., & Kragh-Sorensen, P. (2001). Risk of dementia in Parkinson's disease. A community-based, prospective study. *Neurology*, *56*(6), 730–736.

Abrams, W., Beers, M., & Berkow, R. (1995). Older drivers. In: *Merck Manual of Geriatrics* (Second edition) (p. 1420). Whitehouse Station, NJ: Merck & Company, Inc.

Akiyama, T., Powell, J. L., Mitchell, L. B., Ehlert, F. A., & Baessler, C. (2001). Resumption of driving after life-threatening ventricular tachyarrhythmia. *N. Eng. J. Med.*, *345*(6), 391–397.

Albers, L. J., Hahn, R. K., & Reist, C. (2001). *Handbook of Psychiatric Drugs*. Laguna Hills: Current Clinical Strategies. (pp. 33–49; 67–75).

Aldrich, M. S. (1989). Automobile accidents in patients with sleep disorders. *Sleep*, *12*(6), 487–494.

American Medical Association (1986). *Drug Evaluations* (Sixth edition). Philadelphia: Saunders. pp. 81–110.

Anonymous (2001). *The MS Information Sourcebook*National Multiple Sclerosis Society.

American Psychiatric Association, (1999). *Diagnostic and Statistical Manual of Mental Disorders* (Fourth edition). Washington, DC: American Psychiatric Association.

Babst, D. V., Newman, S., Gordon, N., & Warner, A. (1973). Driving records of methadone maintenance patients in New York State. *J. Drug Issues*, *3*, 285–292.

Ball, K., & Owsley, C. (1991). Identifying correlates of accident involvement for the older driver. *Hum. Factors*, *33*(5), 583–595.

Barbe, P. J., Munoz, A., Findley, L., Anto, J. M., & Agusti, A. G. (1998). Automobile accidents in patients with sleep apnea syndrome. An epidemiological and mechanistic study. *Am. J. Respir. Crit. Care Med.*, *158*(1), 18–22.

Barbone, F., McMahon, A. D., Davey, P. G., Morris, A. D., Reid, I. C., McDevitt, D. O., & MacDonald, T. M. (1998). Association of road-traffic accidents with benzodiazepine use. *Lancet*, *352*(9137), 1331–1336.

Barolin, G. S., & Haslinger, A. (1991). Seizures and driver's license. *Wiener medizinische Wochenschrift Suppl.*, *109*, 9–19.

Beauregard, L. A., Barnard, P. W., Russo, A. M., & Waxman, H. L. (1995). Perceived and actual risks of driving in patients with arrhythmia control devices. *Arch. Intern. Med.*, *155*(6), 609–613.

Bellet, S., Roman, L., Kostis, J., & Slater, A.l. (1968). Continuous electrocardiographic monitoring during automobile driving. *Am. J. Cardiol.*, *22*, 856–862.

Betts, T. (1981). Effects of beta blockade on driving. *Aviat. Space Environ. Med.*, *52*(11 Pt 2), S40–S45.

Blomberg, R. D., & Preusser, D. F. (1974). Narcotic use and driving behavior. *Accid. Anal. Prev.*, *6*, 23–32.

Bloomfield, J. R., Woodworth, G. G., Grant, A. R., Laytohn, T. A., Brown, T. L., McKenzie, D. R., Baker, T. W., & Watson, G. S. (2000). Effects of fexofenadine, diphenhydramine, and alcohol on driving performance. A randomized, placebo-controlled trial in the Iowa driving simulator. *Ann. Intern. Med.*, *132*(5), 354–363.

Borromei, A., Caramelli, R., Chieregatti, G., d'Orsi, U., Guerra, L., Lozito, A., & Vargui, B. (1999). Ability and fitness to drive in Parkinson's disease patients. Functional. *Neurology*, *14*(4), 227–234.

Budd, R. D., Muto, J. J., & Wong, J. K. (1989). Drugs of abuse found in fatally injured drivers in Los Angeles County. *Drug Alcohol Depend.*, *23*, 153–158.

Carr, D. B. (1993). Assessing older drivers for physical and cognitive impairment. *Geriatrics*, *48*, 46–51.

Carr, D. B. (1997). Motor vehicle crashes and drivers with DAT. *Alzheimer Dis. Assoc. Disord.*, *11*(Suppl. 1), 38–41.

Clayton, A. B., Harvey, P. G., & Betts, T. A. (1977). The psychomotor effects of atenolol and other antihistamine agents. *Postgrad. Med. J.*, *53*(3), 157–161.

Cowart, V., & Kandela, P. (1985). Prescription drugs and driving performance. *J. Am. Med. Assoc. (Medical News)*, *254*, 15–27.

Cox, D. J., Clarke, W., Gonder-Frederick, L., & Kovatchev, B. (2001). Driving mishaps and hypoglycemia: Risk and prevention. *Int. J. Clin. Pract.*, *123*, 38–42.

Cox, D. J., Gonder-Frederick, L., & Clarke, W. (1993). Driving performance in Type I diabetes during moderate hypoglycemia. *Diabetes*, *42*(2), 239–243.

Cox, D. J., Gonder-Frederick, L. A., Kovatchev, B. P., Julian, D. M., & Clarke, W. L. (2000). Progressive hypoglycemia's impact on driving simulation performance. Occurrence, awareness and correction. *Diabetes Care*, *23*(2), 163–170.

Crancer, A., & McMurray, L. (1968). Accident and violation rates of Washington's medically restricted drivers. *J. Am. Med. Assoc.*, *205*, 272–276.

Crancer, A., & O'Neall, P. A. (1970). A record analysis of Washington drivers with license restrictions for heart disease. *NW. Med.*, *69*, 409–416.

Curtis, A. B., Conti, J. B., Tucke, K. J., Kubilis, P. S., Reilly, R. E., & Woodward, D. A. (1995). Motor vehicle accidents in patients with an implantable cardioverter-defribillator. *J. Am. Coll. Cardiol.*, *26*(1), 180–184.

DCCT Research Group (1987). Diabetes control and complications trial (DCCT): Results of feasibility study. *Diabetes Care*, *10*, 1–18.

Drachman, D. A., & Swearer, J. M. (1993). Driving and Alzheimer's disease: The risk of crashes. *Neurology*, *43*(12), 2448–2456.

Dubinsky, R. M., Gray, C., Husted, D., Busenbark, K., Vetere-Overfield, B., Wiltfong, D., Parrish, D., & Koller, W. C. (1991). Driving in Parkinson's disease. *Neurology*, *41*(4), 517–520.

Dunn, F. G., Lorimer, A. R., & Lawne, T. D. (1979). Objective measurement of performance during acute stress in patients with essential hypertension: Assessment of the effects of propranolol and metoprolol. *Clin. Sci.*, *57*(Suppl. 5), S413–S415.

Eadington, D. W., & Frier, B. M. (1989). Type I diabetes and driving experience: An eight-year cohort study. *Diabetes Med.*, *6*(2), 137–141.

Edlund, M. J., Conrad, C., & Morris, P. (1989). Accidents among schizophrenic outpatients. *Compr. Psychiatr.*, *30*(6), 522–526.

Ehrlich, E. N. (1991). Diabetes and the license to drive. *Wis. Med. J.*, *90*(3), 115–118.

Evans, L. (1988). Risk of fatality from physical trauma versus sex and age. *J. Trauma*, *28*, 368–378.

Finch, N. J., Leman, R. B., Kratz, J. M., & Gillette, P. C. (1993). Driving safety among patients with automatic cardioverter-defribillators. *J. Am. Med. Assoc.*, *270*(13), 1587–1588.

Findley, L. J., Fabrizio, M. J., Knight, H., Norcross, B. B., LaForte, A. J., & Suratt, P. M. (1989). Driving simulator performance in patients with sleep apnea. *Am. Rev. Respir. Dis.*, *140*(2), 529–530.

Findley, L. J., Levinson, M. P., & Bonnie, R. J. (1992). Driving performance and automobile accidents in patients with sleep apnea. *Clin. Chest Med.*, *13*(3), 427–435.

Fitten, L. J., Perryman, K. M., Wilkinson, C. J., Little, R. J., Burns, M. M., Pachana, N., Mervis, J. R., Malmgren, R., Siembieda, D. W., & Ganzell, S. (1995). Alzheimer and vascular dementias and driving. A prospective road and laboratory study. *J. Am. Med. Assoc.*, *273*(17), 1360–1365.

Fonda, S. J., Wallace, R. B., & Herzog, A. R. (2001). Changes in driving patterns and worsening depressive symptoms among older adults. *J. Gerontol. B. Psychol. Sci. Soc. Sci.*, *56*(6), 343–351.

Francis, J., Martin, D., & Kapoor, W. N. (1990). A prospective study of delirium in hospitalized elderly. *J. Am. Med. Assoc.*, *263*(8), 1097–1101.

Friedland, R. P., Koss, E., Kumar, A., Gaine, S., Metzler, D., Haxby, J. V., & Moore, A. (1988). Motor vehicle crashes in dementia of the Alzheimer type. *Ann. Neurol.*, *24*(6), 782–786.

Frier, B. M., & Wilson, I. M. (1986). Driving after stroke. *Lancet*, *2*(8518), 1280.

Frier, B., Matthews, D. M., Steel, J. M., & Duncan, L. J. (1980). Driving and insulin-dependent diabetes. *Lancet*, *1*(8180), 1232–1234.

Frucht, S., Rogers, J. D., Green, P. E., Gordon, M. F., & Fahn, S. (1999). Falling asleep at the wheel: Motor vehicle mishaps in persons taking pramipexole and ropinirole. *Neurology*, *52*(9), 1908–1910.

Fukushima, Y. (1991). Discussion on the problem of driving license for people with epilepsy. *Jpn. J. Psychiatr. Neurol.*, *45*(2), 333–335.

Gallo, J. J., Rebok, G. W., & Lesikar, S. E. (1999). The driving habits of adults aged 60 years and older. *J. Am. Geriatr. Soc.*, *47*(3), 335–341.

Galski, T., Bruno, R. L., & Ehle, H. T. (1992). Driving after cerebral damage: A model with implications for evaluation. *Am. J. Occup. Ther.*, *46*(4), 324–332.

Galski, T., Bruno, R. L., & Ehle, H. T. (1993). Prediction of behind-the-wheel driving performance in patients with cerebral damage: A discriminant function analysis. *Am. J. Occup. Ther.*, *47*(5), 324–332.

Galski, T., Ehle, H. T., & Bruno, R. L. (1990). Critical assessment of measures to predict outcome of driving evaluations in patients with cerebral damage. *Am. J. Occup. Ther.*, *44*(8), 709–713.

Galski, T., Williams, J. B., & Ehle, H. T. (2000). Effects of opioids on driving ability. *J. Pain Symptom Manag.*, *19*(3), 200–208.

Gengo, F. M., & Manning, C. (1990). A review of the effects of antihistamines on mental processes related to automobile driving. *J. Allergy Clin. Immunol.*, *86*(6), 1034–1039.

Gengo, F., Gabos, C., & Miller, J. K. (1989). The pharmacodynamics of diphenhydramine-induced drowsiness and changes in mental performance. *Clin. Pharmacol. Therapeut.*, *45*(1), 15–21.

Gislason, T., Tomasson, K., Reynisdottir, H., Bjornsson, J. K., & Kristbjarnarson, H. (1997). Medical risk factors amongst drivers in single-car accidents. *J. Int. Med.*, *24*(3), 213–219.

Gordon, N. B. (1976). Influence of narcotic drugs on highway safety. *Accid. Anal. Prev.*, *8*, 3–7.

Grabe, H. J., Wolf, T., Gratz, S., & Laux, G. (1999). The influence of clozapine and typical neuroleptics on information processing of the central nervous system under clinical conditions in schizophrenic disorders: Implications for fitness to drive. *Neuropsychobiology*, *40*(4), 196–201.

Graca, J. (1986). Driving and aging. *Clin. Geriatr. Med.*, *2*, 577–589.

Hansen, G. R. (1999). Loratadine in the high performance aerospace environment. *Aviat. Space Environ. Med.*, *70*(9), 919–924.

Hansotia, P. (1993a). Epilepsy and traffic safety. *Epilepsia*, *34*, 852–858.

Hansotia, P. (1993b). Seizure disorders, diabetes mellitus, and cerebrovascular disease: Considerations for older drivers. *Clin. Geriatr. Med.*, *9*(2), 323–339.

Hansotia, P., & Broste, S. K. (1991). The effect of epilepsy or diabetes mellitus on the risk of automobile accidents. *New Eng. J. Med.*, *324*(1), 22–26.

Harvey, S,C. (1985). Hypnotics and sedatives. In: A. G. Gilman, L. S. Goodman, T. W. Rall, & F. Murad (Eds.), *The Pharmacologic Basis of Therapeutics* (Seventh edition) (pp. 339–371). New York: Macmillan.

Hasegawa, S., Rumnagai, K., & Kaji, S. (1991). Epilepsy and driving: A survey of automobile accidents attributed to seizure. *Jpn. J. Psychiatr. Neurol.*, *45*, 327–331.

Hashimoto, K. (1991). A study on driving status in 98 epileptic patients with driving licenses. *Jpn. J. Psychiatr. Neurol.*, *45*, 323–326.

Hatcher, S., Sims, R., & Thompson, D. (1990). The effects of chronic lithium treatment on psychomotor performance related to driving. *Br. J. Psychiatr.*, *157*, 275–278.

Hauser, R. A., Gauge, rL., Anderson, W. M., & Zesiewicz, T. A. (2000). Pramipexole induced somnolence and episodes of daytime sleep. *Mov. Disord.*, *15*(4), 658–663.

Health Care Financing Administration Office of National Cost Estimates (1988). National health expenditures. *Health Care Financing Review*, *11*(1), 290.

Heikkila, V. M., Korpelainen, J., Turkka, J., Kallanranta, T., & Summala, H. (1999). Clinical evaluation of the driving ability in stroke patients. *Acta Neurol. Scand.*, *99*(6), 349–355.

Heikkila, V. M., Turkka, J., Korpelainen, J., Kallanranta, T., & Summala, H. (1998). Decreased driving ability in people with Parkinson's disease. *J. Neurol. Neurosurg. Psychiatr.*, *64*(3), 325–330.

Hemmelgarn, B., Suissa, S., Huang, A., Boivin, J. F., & Pinard, G. (1997). Benzodiazepine use and the risk of motor vehicle crash in the elderly. *J. Am. Med. Assoc.*, *278*(1), 27–31.

Hindmarch, I. (1986). The effects of psychoactive drugs on car handling and related psychomotor activity. In: J. F. O'Hanlon, & J. J. de Gier (Eds.), *Drugs and Driving* (pp. 71–82). Philadelphia: Taylor and Francis.

Hindmarch, I., & Subhan, Z. (1986). The effects of antidepressants taken with and without alcohol on information processing, psychomotor performance and car handling. In: J. F. O'Hanlon, & J. J. de Gier (Eds.), *Drugs and Driving* (pp. 231–240). Philadelphia: Taylor and Francis.

Hindmarch, I., & Easton, C. (1990). A placebo controlled assessment of mequitazine and astemizole in tests of psychomotor ability. *Int J Clin Pharmacol Res*, *6*(6), 457–464.

Jennings, A. M., Wilson, R. M., & Ward, J. D. (1989). Symptomatic hypoglycemia in NIDDM patients treated with oral hypoglycemic agents. *Diabetes Care*, *12*, 203–208.

John, H. (1980). Hypertension treatment and ability to drive a large vehicle. *Zietschrift fur Gesamte Inn Medizin*, *35*(Suppl. 21), 143–144.

Judd, L. L. (1985). The effect of antipsychotic drugs on driving and driving related psychomotor functions. *Accid. Anal. Prev.*, *17*(4), 319–322.

Kay, G. G., & Harris, A. G. (1999). Loratadine: a non-sedating antihistamine. Review of its effects on cognition, psychomotor performance, mood and sedation. *Clin. Exp. Allergy*, *29*(3), 147–150.

Kay, G. G., & Quig, M. E. (2001). Impact of sedating antihistamines on safety and productivity. *Allergy Asthma Proc.*, *22*(5), 281–283.

Kazniak, A. W., Keyl, P. M., & Albert, M. S. (1991). Dementia and the older driver. *Hum. Factors*, *33*, 527–537.

Kerr, B., Hill, H., Coda, B., Calogero, M., Chapman, C. R., Hunt, E., Buffington, V., & Mackie, A. (1991). Concentration-related effects of morphine on cognition and motor control in human subjects. *Neuropsychopharmacology*, *5*(3), 157–166.

Klavora, P., Heselgrave, R. J., & Young, M. (2000). Driving skills in elderly persons with stroke: Comparison of two new assessment options. *Arch. Phys. Med. Rehabil.*, *81*(6), 701–705.

Koepsell, T. D., Wolf, M. E., McCloskey, L., Buchner, D. M., Wagner, E. H., & Thompson, R. S. (1994). Medical conditions and motor vehicle collision injuries in older adults. *J. Am. Geriatr. Soc.*, *42*(7), 695–700.

Kroenke, K., & Pinholt, E. M. (1990). Reducing polypharmacy in the elderly. A controlled trial of physician feedback. *J. Am. Geriatr. Soc.*, *38*(1), 31–36.

Kurfees, J. F., & Dotson, R. L. (1987). Drug interactions in the elderly. *J. Fam. Pract.*, *25*(5), 477–488.

Laberge-Nadeau, C., Dionne, G., Ekoe, J. M., Hamet, P., Desjardins, D., Messier, S., & Maag, U. (2000). Impact of diabetes on crash risks of truck-permit holders and commercial drivers. *Diabetes Care*, *23*(5), 612–617.

Lachenmayer, L. (2000). Parkinson's disease and the ability to drive. *J. Neurol.*, *247*(Suppl. 4), 28–30.

Larsen, J. P., & Tandberg, E. (2001). Sleep disorders in patients with Parkinson's disease: Epidemiology and management. *Cent. Nerv. Syst. Drugs*, *15*(4), 267–275.

Larsen, B., Otto, H., Dorsecheid, E., & Larsen, R. (1999). Effects of long-term opioid therapy on psychomotor function in patients with cancer pain or non-malignant pain. *Anaesthesist*, *48*(9), 613–624.

Laubichler, W. (1992). The driver's license and epilepsy. *Blutalkohol*, *29*(2), 139–146.

Legh-Smith, J., Wade, D. T., & Hewer, R. L. (1986). Driving after stroke. *J. Roy. Soc. Med.*, *79*(4), 200–203.

Lings, S., & Dupont, E. (1992). Driving with Parkinson's disease. A controlled laboratory investigation. *Acta Neurol. Scand.*, *88*(1), 33–39.

Lings, S., & Jensen, P. B. (1991). Driving after stroke: a controlled laboratory investigation. *Int. Disabil. Stud.*, *13*(3), 74–82.

Linnoila, M., Guthrie, S., & Lister, R. (1986). Mechanisms of drug-induced impairment of driving. In: J. F. O'Hanlon, & J. J. de Gier (Eds.), *Drugs and Driving* (pp. 29–50). Philadelphia: Taylor and Francis.

Lucas-Blaustein, M. J., Filipp, L., Dungan, C., & Tune, L. (1988). Driving in patients with dementia. *J. Am. Geriatr. Soc.*, *36*, 1087–1092.

Marottoli, R. A., Mendes de Leon, C. F., Glass, T. A., Williams, C. S., Cooney, L. M., Berkman, L. F., & Tinetti, M. E. (1997). Driving cessation and increased depressive symptoms: Prospective evidence from the New Haven EPESE. *J. Am. Geriatr. Soc.*, *45*, 202–206.

Masa, J. F., Rubio, M., & Findley, L. J. (2000). Habitually sleepy drivers have a high frequency of automobile crashes associated with respiratory disorders during sleep. *Am. J. Respir. Crit. Care Med.*, *162*(4 Pt 1), 1407–1412.

McGwin, G., Sims, R. V., Pulley, L., & Roseman, J. M. (2000). Relations among chronic medical conditions, medications, and automobile crashes in the elderly: A population-based case-control study. *Am. J. Epidemiol.*, *152*(5), 424–431.

Meijler, W. J. (2000). Driving ban for patients on chronic opioid therapy unfounded. *Nederlands Tijdscrift Voor Geneeskunde*, *144*(34), 1644–1645.

Meltzer, E. O. (1990). Performance effects on antihistamines. *J. Allergy Clin. Immunol.*, *86*(4), 613–619.

Menzin, J., Lang, K. M., Levy, P., & Levy, E. (2000). A general model of the effects of sleep medications on the risk and cost of motor vehicle accidents and its application in France. *Pharmacoeconomics*, *19*(1), 69–78.

Miranda, M., Diaz, V., Venegas, P., & Villagra, R. (2001). Sleepiness attacks while driving: adverse effects of new antiparkinson's drugs. *Revista Medica de Chile*, *129*(5), 585–586.

Moeller, T. P. (1989). Sensory changes in the elderly. *Dent. Clin. N. Am.*, *33*(1), 23–31.

Moeller, J., & Mathiowetz, N. (1989). Prescribed medicines: A summary of use and expenditures by Medicare beneficiaries (DHHS Publication No. PHS 89-3448). *National Medical Expenditure Survey Research Findings 3, National center for Health Services Research and Health Care Technology Assessment*, Rockville, MD: Public Health Service.

Mola, S. (1995). Neurological diseases and driving. *Rev. Neurol.*, *23*(120), 334–350.

Moller, H. (2001). Antiparkinsonian drugs and "sleep attacks". *Can. Med. Assoc. J.*, *164*(7), 1038–1039.

Moller, J. C., Stiasny, K., Cassel, W., Peter, J. H., Kruger, H. P., & Oertel, W. H. (2000). "Sleep attacks" in Parkinson's patients. A side effect of nonergoline dopamine agonists or a class effect of dopamine agonists? *Der Nervenartz*, *71*(8), 670–676.

Mortimer, J. A. (1983). Alzheimer's disease and senile dementia: Prevalence and incidence. In: B. Reisberg (Ed.), *Alzheimer's disease* (pp. 141–148). New York: Free Press.

Mortimer, R. G., & Howat, P. A. (1986). Effects of alcohol and diazepam, singly and in combination, on some aspects of driving performance. In: J. F. O'Hanlon, & J. J. de Gier (Eds.), *Drugs and Driving* (pp. 163–178). Philadelphia: Taylor and Francis.

Murray, J. B. (1984). Effects of valium and librium on human psychomotor and cognitive functions. *Genet. Psychol. Monogr.*, *109*(2D half), 167–197.

Nagi, S. Z. (1976). An epidemiology of disability among adults in the United States. *Milbank Memorial Fund Quarterly*, *54*, 439–468.

Naughton, T. J., Pepler, R. D., & Walker, J. (1982). Investigate road accident risklevels for heart attack (myocardial infarction) victims. *Final Report on NHT SA Contract No DTNH-22-80-C-07325.* Darien, CT: Dunlap and Associates, Inc.

Niveau, G., & Kelley-Puskas, M. (2001). Psychiatric disorders and fitness to drive. *J. Med. Ethics*, *27*(1), 36–39.

Novak, A. J. (1991). Driving and epilepsy: The effects of medication. *J. Am. Med. Assoc.*, *265*(22), 2961–2962.

Ondo, W. G., Dat Wong, K., Khan, H., Atasi, F., Kwak, C., & Jankovic, J. (2001). Daytime sleepiness and other sleep disorders in Parkinson's disease. *Neurology*, *57*(8), 1392–1396.

Organization for Economic Cooperation and Development (OECD) (1985). *Traffic Safety of Elderly Road Users.* Paris: OECD.

Owsley, C., Ball, K., Sloane, M. E., Roenker, D. L., & Bruni, J. R. (1991). Visual/cognitive correlates of vehicle accidents in older drivers. *Psychol. Aging*, *6*, 403–415.

Owsley, C., Stalvey, B., Wells, J., & Sloane, M. E. (1999). Older drivers and cataract: driving habits and crash risk. *J. Gerontol.*, *54*(4), M203–MM211.

O'Hanlon, J. F., & Ramaekers, J. G. (1995). Antihistamine effects on actual driving performance in a standard test: A summary of Dutch experience, 1989–94. *Allergy*, *50*(3), 234–242.

O'Hanlon, J. F., Robbe, H. W., Vermeeren, A., van Leeuwen, C., & Danjou, P. E. (1998). Venlafaxine's effects on healthy volunteer's driving, psychomotor, and vigilance performance during 15-day fixed and incremental dosing regimens. *J. Clin. Psychopharmacol.*, *18*(3), 212–221.

O'Hanlon, J. F., & Volkerts, E. R. (1986). Hypnotics and actual driving performance. *Acta Psychiatr. Scand. Suppl.*, *332*, 95–104.

Pals, S., Bhattacharya, K. F., Agapito, C., & Chauahuri, K.R. (2001). A study of excessive daytime sleepiness and its clinical significance in three groups of Parkinson's disease patients taking pramipexole, cabergoline and levodopa mono and combination therapy. *J. Neural Transm.*, *108*(1), 71–77.

Palva, E. S., Linnoila, M., Routledge, P., & Seppala, T. (1982). Actions and interactions of diazepam and alcohol on psychomotor skills in young and middle-aged subjects. *Acta Pharmacol. Toxicol. (Copenhagen)*, *50*(5), 363–369.

Panizza, D., & Lecasble, M. (1985). Effects of atenolol on car drivers in a prolonged stress situation. *Eur. J. Clin. Pharmacol.*, *28*, 97–99.

Partyka, S. C. (1983). *Comparison by Age of Drivers in Two-Car Fatal Crashes.* Washington, DC: National Highway Traffic Safety Administration.

Philpot, E. E. (2000). Safety of second generation antihistamines. *Allergy Asthma Proc.*, *21*(1), 15–20.

Polen, M. R., & Friedman, G. D. (1988). Automobile injury – Selected risk factors and prevention in the health care setting. *J. Am. Med. Assoc.*, *259*, 77–80.

Popkin, C. L., & Waller, P. F. (1988). Epilepsy and driving in North Carolina: An exploratory study. In: *32nd Annual Proceedings of the Association for the Advancement of Automotive Medicine* (pp. 347–358). Des Plaines, IL.

Ray, W. A., Fought, R. I., & Decker, M. D. (1992). Psychoactive drugs and the risk of injurious motor vehicle crashes in elderly drivers. *Am. J. Epidemiol.*, *136*(7), 873–883.

Ray, W. A., Gurwitz, J., Decker, M. D., & Kennedy, D. L. (1992). Medications and the safety of the older driver: Is there a basis for concern? *Hum. Factors*, *34*(1), 33–47.

Ray, W. A., Thapa, P. B., & Sho, rR. I. (1993). Medications and the older driver. *Clin. Geriatr. Med.*, *9*(2), 413–438.

Regestein, Q. R. (1984). Treatment of insominia in the elderly. In: C. Salzman (Ed.), *Clinical Geriatric Psychopharmacology* (pp. 149–170). New York: McGraw-Hill.

Reidel, D. B., Quasten, R., Hausen, C., & O'Hanlon, J. F. (1988). *A study comparing the hypnotic efficacies and residual effects on actual driving performance of midazolam 15 mg, triazolam 0.5 mg, temazepam 20 mg, and placebo in shiftworkers on night duty.* Maastricht, the Netherlands: Institute for Drugs, Safety and Behavior.

Reidenberg, M. M., Levy, M., Warne, r. H., Coutinho, C. B., Schwartz, M. A., Yu, G., & Cheripko, J. (1978). Relationship between diazepam dose, plasma level,age, and central nervous system depression. *Clin. Pharmacol. Ther., 23*(4), 371–374.

Retchin, S. M. (1989). Using a severity of illness model for predicting driving capabilities for older drivers. Paper presented at National Institute on Ageing/National Highway Traffic Safety Administration Workshop, *Research and Development Needed to Improve Safety and Mobility of Older Persons*, Bethesda, MD.

Retchin, S. M., & Anapolle, J. (1983). An overview of the older driver. *Clin. Geriatr. Med., 9,* 279–296.

Reuben, D. B., Silliman, R. A., & Traines, M. (1988). The aging driver. Medicine, policy and ethics. *J. Am. Geriatr. Soc., 36*(12), 1135–1142.

Rizzo, M., McGhee, D. V., Dawson, J. D., & Anderson, S. N. (2001). Simulated car crashes at intersections in drivers with Alzheimer's disease. *Alzheimer Dis. Assoc. Disord., 15*(1), 10–20.

Rizzo, M., Reinach, S., McGhee, D., & Dawson, J. (1997). Simulated car crashes and crash predictors in drivers with Alzheimer's disease. *Arch. Neurol., 54*(5), 545–551.

Robbe, H. W., & O'Hanlon, J. F. (1995). Acute and subchronic effects of paroxetine 20 and 40 mg on actual driving, psychomotor performance and subjective assessments in healthy volunteers. *Eur. Neuropsychopharmacol., 5*(1), 35–42.

Salzman, C. (1985). Geriatric psychopharmacology. *Annual Review of Medicine, 36,* 217–228.

Salzman, C. (1984). Pharmacokinetics of psychotropic drugs and the aging process. In: C. Salzman (Ed.), *Clinical Geriatric Psychopharmacology* (pp. 32–45). New York: McGraw-Hill.

Schacter, S. C. (1998). Iatrogenic seizures. *Neurol. Clin., 16*(1), 157–170.

Schlosberg, A. (1990). Traffic violations in schizophrenics before and after hospitalization. *Harefuah, 119*(10), 307–308.

Schultheis, M. T., Garay, E., & DeLuca, J. (2001). The influence of cognitive impairment on driving performance in multiple sclerosis. *Neurology, 56*(8), 1089–1094.

Seppala, T., Linnoila, M., & Mattila, M. J. (1979). Drugs, alcohol and driving. *Drugs, 17*(5), 389–408.

Seppala, T., Mattila, M. J., Palva, E. S., & Aranko, K. (1986). Combined effects of anxiolytics and alcohol on psychomotor performance in young and middle-aged subjects. In: J. F. O'Hanlon, & J. J. de Gier (Eds.), *Drugs and Driving* (pp. 179–190). Philadelphia: Taylor and Francis.

Settipane, R. A. (1999). Complications of allergic rhinitis. *Allergy Asthma Proc., 20*(4), 9–213.

Sims, R. V., Owsley, C., Allman, R. M., Ball, K., & Smoot, T. M. (1998). A preliminary assessment of the medical and functional factors associated with vehicle crashes by older adults. *J. Am. Geriatr. Soc., 46,* 556–561.

Sjogren, P., Banning, A. M., Christensen, C. B., & Pederson, O. (1994). Continuous reaction time after single dose, long-term oral and epidural opioid administration. *Eur. J. Anaesthesiol., 11*(2), 95–100.

Skegg, D. C. G., Richards, S. M., & Doll, R. (1979). Minor tranquilizers and road accidents. *Br. Med. J., 1*(6168), 917–919.

Songer, T. J., LaPorte, R. E., Dorman, J. S., Orchard, T. J., Cruickshanks, K. J., Becker, D. J., & Drash, A. L. (1988). Motor vehicle accidents and IDDM. *Diabetes Care, 11*(9), 701–707.

Soyka, M., Dittert, S., Gartenmeier, A., & Schafer, M. (1998). Driving fitness in therapy with antidepressive drugs. *Versicherungsmedizin, 50*(2), 59–66.

Spira, N., Dysken, M. W., Lazarus, L. W., Davis, J. M., & Salzman, C. (1984). Treatment of agitation and psychosis. In: C. Salzman (Ed.), *Clinical Geriatric Psychopharmacology* (pp. 49–76). New York: McGraw-Hill.

Stahl, S. M. (1998). Basic psychopharmacology of antidepressants. *J. Clin. Psychiatr., 59*(Suppl. 4), 5–14.

Starmer, G. A. (1986). A review of the effects of analgesics on driving performance handling. In: J. F. O'Hanlon, & J. J. de Gier (Eds.), *Drugs and Driving* (pp. 251–270). Philadelphia: Taylor and Francis.

Terry, R., & Katzman, R. (1983). Senile dementia of the Alzheimer's type: Defining a disease. In: R. Katzman, & B. R. Terry (Eds.), *The Neurology of Ageing* (pp. 51–84). Philadelphia: FA Davis.

Thomas, R. E. (1998). Benzodiazepine use and motor vehicle accidents. Systematic review of reported association. *Can. Fam. Physician, 44,* 799–808.

Trappe, H. J., Wenzlaff, P., & Grellman, G. (1998). Should patients with implantable cardioverter-defribillators be allowed to drive? Observations in 291 patients from a single center over an 11-year period. *J. Intervent. Card. Electrophysiol., 2*(2), 193–201.

Trobe, J. D., Waller, P. F., Cook-Flannagan, C. A., Teshima, S. M., & Bieliauskas, L. (1996). Crashes and violations among drivers with Alzheimer's disease. *Arch. Neurol., 53*(5), 411–416.

Vainio, A., Ollilia, J., Matikainen, E., Rosenberg, P., & Kalso, E. (1995). Driving ability in cancer patients receiving long-term morphine analgesia. *Lancet, 346,* 667–670.

Van Laar, M. W., van Willigenburg, A. P., & Volkert, E. R. (1995). Acute and subchronic effects of nefazodone and imipramine on highway driving, cognitive functions, and daytime sleepiness in healthy adult and elderly subjects. *J. Clin. Psychopharmacol., 15*(1), 30–40.

Veneman, F. (1996). Diabetes mellitus and traffic accidents. *Neth. J. Med., 48*(1), 24–28.

Vermeeren, A., & O'Hanlon, J. F. (1998). Fexofenadine's effects, alone and with alcohol, on actual driving and psychomotor performance. *J. Investig. Allergol. Clin. Immunol., 101*(3), 306–311.

Wallace, R. B., & Retchin, S. M. (1992). A geriatric and gerontologic perspective on the effects of medical conditions on older drivers: Discussion of Waller. *Hum. Factors, 34*(1), 17–24.

Waller, J. A. (1965). Chronic medical conditions and traffic safety: A review of California Experience. *New Eng. J. Med., 273,* 1413–11420.

Waller, J. A. (1967). Cardiovascular disease, ageing, and traffic accidents. *J. Chron. Dis., 20,* 615–620.

Waller, P. E. (1985). Preventing injury to the elderly. *Aging and Public Health* (pp. 103–146) Springer.

Waller, J. A. (1992). Research and other issues concerning effects of medical conditions on elderly drivers. *Hum. Factors, 34*(1), 3–15.

Waller, J., & Goo, J. T. (1969). Highway crash and citation patterns and chronic medical conditions. *J. Safety Res., 1,* 13–27.

Willumeit, H. P., Ott, H., Neurbert, W., Hemmerling, K. G., Schratzer, M., & Fichte, K. (1984). Alcohol interaction of lormetazepam, mepindolol sulphate and diazepam measured by performance on the driving simulator. *Pharmacopsychiatry, 7*(2), 36–43.

Wylie, K. R., Thompson, D. J., & Wildgust, H. J. (1993). Effects of depot neuroleptics on driving performance in chronic schizophrenic patients. *J. Neurol. Neurosurg. Psychiatr., 56*(8), 910–913.

Zacny, J. P. (1995). A review of the effects of opioids on psychomotor and cognitive functioning in humans. *Exp. Clin. Psychopharmacol., 3,* 432–466.

van Zomeren, A. H., Brouwer, W. H., & Minderhoud, J. M. (1987). Acquired brain damage and driving: A review. *Arch. Phys. Med. Rehabil., 68*(10), 697–705.

10

DRIVING AND THE LAW

THOMAS GALSKI AND MARY ANNE McDONALD

Driving is often regarded as a right, or entitlement in American society. However, it is a privilege granted by States to help individual citizens in their pursuit of life, liberty and happiness, a privilege that, in light of States' responsibility to ensure the health, safety, and welfare of its entire citizenry must be balanced against the public's rights to reasonable safety and protection from actual or potential dangers as, for example, from drivers whose impairments can compromise driving safely (State v Zoppi, 196 NJ Super 596, Law Div, 1984; DMV v Granziel, 236 NJ Super 191, App Div, 1989).

As summarized in a recent article by Galski et al. (2000), a person can exercise this privilege while, simultaneously, the public interest is protected when and if a person can successfully demonstrate driving competence to the State. Typically, the Division of Motor Vehicles (DMV), or the equivalent agency, empowered by the State has the responsibility and legal authority to decide on licensure. DMVs are guided by and must follow licensing statutes and regulations that describe eligibility and procedures for obtaining a driver's license. Generally, States require that drivers qualify themselves by passing physical, written, and behind-the-wheel tests regarded as valid measures of real-world driving safety. These tests usually include measures of visual acuity (e.g., 20/50 vision), practical knowledge (e.g., stopping distances at various speeds), operational ability (e.g., steering, lane use, turning, parking), and responses to traffic control devices (e.g., stopping at stop signs).

Drivers usually provide evidence of their capacity to safely operate a motor vehicle only once to the licensing authority; this typically happens at 16 or 17-years old when a person has presumably attained sufficient physical and mental maturity to be entrusted with the responsibilities of driving. After successful completion of the examination and award of a permanent license, drivers do not generally require reexaminations throughout adult life, only renewals of licensure; renewal procedures, which occur at intervals of 2–12 years in States throughout the country, most commonly involve a check for revocations or suspensions with payment of appropriate fees and can be done in the majority of States electronically or by mail. However, if and when States believe that a person's fitness to drive is in doubt because of reports by police and others, a history of accidents or violations, appearance or demeanor at renewal, and mental or physical impairments, a number of means are available to ensure the community's safety. For example, States can deny, withdraw or restrict a person's driving privilege; compel a retaking of standard licensing tests; shorten renewal intervals; insist on personal rather than electronic or mail renewal in order to evaluate appearance and demeanor; and, require mental and/or physical examinations.

While there are some common aspects regarding legal procedures of licensure, it is evident that much variability exists from State to State. As such, the purpose of this chapter is to provide an overview of these differences to increase the reader's awareness of the various aspects of clinical driving evaluation that can be impacted by legal issues. While in many States physicians are held responsible for reporting any driving-related impairments to the State, in practice driving concerns are seen at various stages of treatment for individuals with neurological compromise. As such, concerns regarding reporting impaired drivers is not limited to physician alone, but are commonly raised by other clinicians, such as psychologist and occupational therapists. To this end, our goal is to provide information to clinicians at all level, as well as family members of individuals with neurological compromise.

DEFINING MEDICAL CONDITIONS: FOCUS OF DRIVING LAW

Every State has sought to identify and regulate the license eligibility of unsafe drivers; these efforts have historically focused on conditions that affect consciousness, physical ability and coordination, particularly epilepsy, cardiovascular (e.g., stroke, diabetes), and neurological conditions (e.g., brain injury). Perhaps based on the number of studies in recent decades revealing elevated risk of crashes and traffic violations in people with various other medical conditions, diseases, impairments or frailties (e.g., diabetes, hypoglycemia, visual disturbances, sleep disorders, Parkinson's disease, dementia, and age-related cognitive impairments), many States have expanded the historically limited range of conditions considered in laws ands statutes (Waller, 1965, 1967; Crancer & McMurray, 1968; Waller & Goo, 1969; Crancer & O'Neall, 1970; Frier et al., 1980; Popkin & Waller, 1988; Friedland et al., 1988; Aldrich, 1989; Hansotia & Broste, 1991; Owsley et al., 1991; Hemmelgarn et al., 1997; Gallo et al., 1999; Laberge-Nadeau et al., 2000; Masa et al., 2000; Aarsland et al., 2001).

For example, New York focuses on loss of consciousness (LOC) defined as "the condition of not being aware of one's surroundings or of one's existence and the inability to receive, interpret or react to sensory impressions as the result of epilepsy, syncope, cataplexy, narcolepsy and other disorders affecting consciousness or control" (New York Comprehensive Codes, Rules and Regulations, Title 15, Section 9.2a). Similarly, Arizona regulations define alterations in consciousness as "sudden and unanticipated partial or complete loss of awareness ... partial or complete loss of mental contact with the environment ... sudden confusion ... or the sudden inability to recollect immediate events" (Arizona Administrative Code Regulations 17-4-522 A1). New Jersey statutes describe a safe driver as a person "free from recurrent convulsive seizures ... recurrent periods of impaired consciousness or from impairment or loss of motor coordination for a period of one year ... with or without medication, and ... physically qualified to operate a motor vehicle" (New Jersey Administrative Code 13:19-4.1-5.10). Nevada regulations describe conditions that can cause a lapse of consciousness, including "epilepsy, diabetes, frequently reoccurring fainting or dizzy spells caused by major medical problems and major head injuries" (Nevada Administrative Code, Chapter 483.330).

Other States regulations, such as Maryland, center on medical conditions affected by actual or potential LOC, such as cardiovascular impairments marked by recurrent lapses of consciousness, diseases of the nervous system, including cerebral hemorrhage or infarction, and traumatic brain injury which have resulted in a significant change in personality, alertness or ability to make decisions (Code of Maryland Regulations 11.17.03.04). Michigan centers on conditions which "cause or contribute to a lapse of consciousness, blackout, seizure, fainting spell, syncope or other impairment of the level of consciousness ... an impairment of driving judgment or reaction time ... a violent or aggressive action relating to the operation of a motor vehicle" (Michigan Administrative Code, Regulations 257.851).

Similarly, Pennsylvania cites epilepsy as the primary condition but adds other physical and medical conditions that subject a driver to denial or recall of licensure, including loss or impairment of limbs resulting in functional limitation, unstable diabetes or hypoglycemia, cerebral vascular insufficiency or cardiac disease, periodic LOC or awareness regardless of cause, mental deficiency, mental or emotional disorders of organic or functional etiology, use of drugs or substances that can impair driving skill regardless even if prescribed medically, and any other condition that could interfere with ability to operate a motor vehicle in the opinion of an examining physician (75 Pa Stat 1518).

In sum, the type of medical conditions considered detrimental to driving that require reporting to the State vary significantly. Not only there is a difference in what conditions States recognize, but also in how those conditions are defined and what specific aspects of that condition are deemed detrimental. This is best exemplified by considering the varying definitions of "loss of consciousness" (LOC); while some States such as NY provide a specific definition and list medical conditions that LOC results from (e.g., epilepsy, narcolepsy), other states only provide a global definition. Similarly, some States such as NJ, include a time interval (i.e., no LOC for period of 1 year), while many States do not include this specific requirement and do not provide temporal guidelines.

The challenge to the clinician faced with making determination of driving capacity is in being knowledgeable about the specific State he/she is practicing in. Given the great variability, it would be impossible to make general guidelines or recommendations. However, to help begin to highlight some of these points, we have compiled a state-by-state table summarizing some key aspects of reporting and license requirements and license renewal information (see Appendix A). The table provides a brief referred to their individual State departments to obtain a full copy of the States requirements.

EVALUATION OF DRIVING CAPACITY

The scientific literature contains a basic and expanding compendium of impairments related to driving performance, including but not limited to sensory deficiencies (e.g., defects in visual and auditory acuity, glare and contrast sensitivity), motoric problems (e.g., loss or reduction in strength, coordination and reaction time), and cognitive impairments (e.g., poor visual scanning of traffic and environment, problems in spatial perception, difficulties in attention and concentration) (Gurgold & Harden, 1978; Sivak et al., 1981; Evans & Ginsburg, 1985; Hopewell & van Zomeren, 1990; Galski et al., 1992; Galski et al., 1993; Ball et al., 1993; Schultheis et al., 2001). There are, however, no national, State, or industry standards for evaluating drivers, no normative data relevant to a person's performance on which to base pass–fail decisions, and no established guidelines for interpretation of results. Additionally, there is no pattern of neurological, perceptual, cognitive, or motoric impairments that consistently renders a person with one or more medical conditions unfit to drive (Galski et al., 2000).

Nevertheless, physicians are viewed by the law as the authorities in evaluating the fitness to drive of individuals whose capacity to safely operate a motor vehicle may be compromised by medical disease or disorders. Physicians recognize the centrality of their role in the licensing process, namely, identification of the at-risk driver while maintaining standards of medical practice and adhering to sound ethical and legal practices in collaboration with patients, families, State and agencies (Fitten, 1997; Kakaiya et al., 2000).

In a report on impaired drivers and their physicians by the American Medical Association's Council on Ethical and Judicial Affairs (1999), physicians were found to have an ethical responsibility to assess patients' physical and mental impairments that could adversely affect driving abilities. At the same time, the report declared that there are "few clear-cut standards or valid measures to assess driving competency at physicians' immediate disposal" and, therefore, properly referred responsibility for actual determination of driving fitness to States' licensing bodies (e.g., DMVs, Department of Public Safety).

Despite ongoing debate, this ethical responsibility has carried over to legal responsibilities, as illustrated by past legal cases. For example, failure to advice individuals about the impact of their medical conditions (including medications) on driving ability has been deemed negligent behaviors (Freese v Lemmon, 1973; Gooden v Tips, 1983; Wilshinsky v Medina, 1989). Furthermore, previous cases have demonstrated that physicians can be held liable for their patient's car crash and for third-party injuries caused by their patients because of failure to advice their patients about potential driving impairment resulting from their medical condition or medications (Duvall v Goldin, 1984; Calwall v Hassan, 1996).

Notably, although physicians and other clinicians are deemed responsible for the identification of potential at-risk drivers, most States require a substantive evaluation before action is taken to deny, restrict, suspend, or revoke a license (or to reinstate a license). This procedure for the evaluation of driving capacity in the identified at-risk driver varies widely among the States. Furthermore, in many cases the parties making the determination about fitness to safely operate a motor vehicle are often persons who hold the same or similar administrative and professional positions in the various states. These decision-makers are generally personnel in the State's licensing body who are often assisted in their duties by an independent medical advisory board comprised of physicians and, in some states, non-medical members. Information used in determinations generally consists of physician reports and statements, including information about medical conditions, relationship of medical conditions to driving ability, treatments and medications, and record of accidents and violations.

New York's process of evaluating fitness to drive is similar to that in other states (e.g., see District of Columbia Municipal Regulations, Title 18, Section 106; Kansas Administrative Regulations 92-52-11; Nevada Administrative Code, Chapter 483, Section 330; New Jersey Administrative Code 13:19-5.1). Specific regulations apply to applicants for drivers' licenses who have ever suffered LOC, licensees who have suffered LOC since their last licenses were issued, persons who must submit physician statements as a condition for continued licensing, and licensees about whom evidence of lost consciousness has been received by the Commissioner of the Department of Motor Vehicles (New York Comprehensive Codes, Rules and Regulations, Title 15, Section 9.1).

In addition to these legal procedures, many physicians will refer patients to clinical driver evaluations, upon identification of an at-risk driver. The evaluations (covered in Chapters 1 and 2) can provide greater information about the individual's driving capacity and often work in conjunction with the States DMV and Medical Boards.

Persons who are subject to these regulations may be deemed fit for licensing if certain conditions are met (e.g., no LOC within prior 12 months) and confirmed by a physician's statement. In certain cases (e.g., LOC due solely to a change in medication directed by a physician), the Commissioner may disagree with or question the physician's statement after the recommendation of the Commissioner's medical consultant (New York Comprehensive Codes, Rules and Regulations, Title 15, Section 9.3a–c). Licensing of a person who has experienced a LOC but is fit to drive may be conditioned on submission of periodic physicians' statements when the submitting physician or the medical consultant to the Commissioner opines that they are necessary or desirable (New York Comprehensive Codes, Rules and Regulations, Title 15, Section 9.5). Once again, how these limitations or restrictions are decided and implemented vary from State to State.

For example, in Maine, the Secretary of State requires drivers to provide a medical report when information has been received concerning the existence of a medical condition that may affect driving ability (Code of Maine Regulations 29–250, Chapter 3, Section 2C). If the medical report is not provided, or indicates that the driver is not competent to operate a motor vehicle, the Secretary of State may obtain advice from the medical advisory board, or one of its members; require a driving evaluation; conduct a hearing; and suspend driving privileges (Code of Maine Regulations 29–250, Chapter 3, Section 2D).

Interestingly, Maine has developed *Functional Ability Profiles* for use by the medical advisory board in guiding decisions for persons with head injury, stroke, neurological, and related musculoskeletal conditions (Code of Maine Regulations 29–250, Chapter 3, Section 2). Basically, the *Functional Ability Profile* includes categories of disorders or impairments (e.g., hearing loss/vertigo, head injury, neurological conditions, psychiatric disorders, cardiovascular disorders). Each category is rated by presence/absence of medical condition(s), degree of recovery or compensation, and extent of active impairment (minimal, mild, moderate, or severe) and developed into an estimate of general functional ability; recommendations as to licensing action and periodic review emanate from these estimates. For example, a head injury patient with minimal active impairment may be recommended for no driving license restrictions, but a head injury patient with severe impairment marked by significant deficits and no potential for improvement may be prohibited from driving.

Additionally, Illinois has created a helpful framework for use by their medical advisory board in determining fitness to drive based on estimates of drivers' cognitive functioning, mental and physical condition(s), and measures of vision obtained by screening. Specifically, Illinois takes into account a person's emotional and intellectual ability to operate a motor vehicle: (a) freedom from distractions of hallucinations, impulsive behavior, homicidal and/or suicidal tendencies associated with any medical condition; (b) orientation, including the ability to prepare destination in advance of actual driving; (c) recognition and understanding of symbols or language and road signs with ability to see objects in field of vision, recognize their significance and react to them with sufficient speed; (d) possession of sufficient memory to recall destination and significance of road signs and hazards as well as operational control of vehicle; and (e) ability to distinguish left from right, judge distance and relative speed of own vehicle and other vehicles. Moreover, it considers a person's motor and sensory abilities: (f) ability to sit in a stable and erect posture; (g) ability to turn head at east

25 degrees in either direction; (h) ability to control the vehicle by grip steering wheel, reaching controls and pedals with ease and without unbalancing or stressing the driver; (i) ability to perform routine operations of vehicle with steady, coordinated movements in average reaction time and unimpeded by muscle, joint or skeletal deformity; (j) ability to sustain consciousness throughout driving interval; and (k) freedom from severe pain which could cause incapacitation or inability to control the vehicle.

NOTIFICATION OF THE LICENSING AUTHORITY

The manner in which a driver's health status or injury comes to the attention of licensing authorities varies among the states. Alternatives include self-reporting by the driver and reporting by law enforcement officials often related to the occurrence of an accident, physicians or other health care providers usually associated with onset or deterioration in a medical condition, and others, including family members and neighbors with a concern about a driver's ability to safely operate a vehicle.

In terms of self-reporting, States typically require drivers to notify the licensing authority of any medical conditions that could adversely affect driving only when applying for or renewing a license. Pertinent questions are usually presented on license and renewal applications and drivers are expected to answer all questions completely and truthfully. The situation is less clear with medical occurrences between license renewals or required periodic reports in cases of patients already known to licensing authorities because of a medical condition. Many people, out of ignorance or in an effort to avoid the possibility of lost or restricted licensure, may not report themselves at these times. The failure to self-report may have unfortunate consequences since individuals who drive without the State's knowledge of their medical condition may run an increased risk of civil or criminal liability and/or loss of insurance coverage in the event of an accident. For example, Jacobs (1978) noted that, because responsibility for an accident will probably be assigned to one of the involved drivers, a driver who fails to report a medical condition may have the difficult problem of proving the condition was not the cause of the accident and incur costly court judgments and awards from an injured party for pain and suffering, permanent disability, extended hospitalization, and lost wages for negligence, even in States with no-fault insurance.

With respect to reporting by physicians, few States require the reporting of any medical conditions that may jeopardize safety of the driver or public; the majority of States provide physicians with an opportunity to report on a permissive basis (Pidikiti & Novack, 1991; Malinowski & Petrucelli, 1997; Reuben et al., 1998). However, six States – California, Delaware, Nevada, New Jersey, Oregon, and Pennsylvania – currently have mandatory reporting laws regarding potentially unsafe drivers. While the exact terms of these provisions vary by State, they generally assert that any physician who diagnoses or treats a person with a disease or disorder listed in the regulations must report the person's name, age, and address to a central state agency, usually the Department of Motor Vehicles or Department of Public Safety. The variations in the requirements generally involve the circumstances under which persons must be reported, such as all persons with an identified condition (e.g., epilepsy) or only those whose condition interferes with ability to drive; whether the intended use of the information is specified; and, the penalty, if any, for failing to report.

Other laws may require physicians, as part of proper medical care and management, to provide patients with warning and counseling in these matters. Expanding legal opinion suggests that physicians may be held liable for failing to provide proper care in the absence of specific warnings about potential adverse effects of their patients' medical condition or treatment on driving. Moreover, physicians who have taken charge of a patient's care have an obligation with the weight of legal duty to protect potential victims or classes of victims (i.e., public) from any foreseeable danger or harm that may emanate from the patient's condition or treatment. This obligation arises out of the assumption that the physician knows or should know a patient's dangerous propensities with a reasonable degree of medical certainty by virtue of superior knowledge and unique position in the person's life (Tarasoff v Regents of University of California, 17 Cal 3d 425, Sup Ct, 1976; Antrim & Engum, 1989; Bor, 1990). Case law has shown that physicians can be held liable for negligently failing to warn (Freese v Lemmon, 210 NW 2d 576, Iowa, 1973; Gooden v Tips, 651 SW 2d 364, Tex App Tyler, 1983; Naidu v Laird, 539 A 2d 1064, Del Sup, 1988; Galski et al., 2000).

Whether there is permissive or mandatory reporting, experience, and anecdotal evidence suggest that physicians often do not report patients with medical conditions that may adversely affect driving safety. Under-reporting may be related to physicians' belief that inaction relieves them of actual or potential liability, reluctance to put patients through a time-consuming and costly driving evaluation if confident in their clinical procedures and medical history to determine driver safety, concern about potential suits for defamation of character, and hesitancy to assume responsibility to report if the State does not require it (Pierce, 1993).

Additionally, non-reporting may be related to physicians' poor knowledge of relevant laws, medical restrictions and practices, as exemplified in several recent studies. Specifically, King et al. (1992) found that 400 physicians in general practice and 246 hospital-based physicians surveyed by questionnaire demonstrated significant weakness in knowledge of laws and the basis for making sound recommendations about fitness to drive. In 1997, Mclachlan discovered variability in attitude and practice of reporting various medical conditions by neurologists who, perhaps more than other medical specialists, are regularly involved in the care and treatment of patients with disorders that can affect driving safety. Interestingly, seizure disorders were reported more often than other medical conditions; however, only 50% of physicians reported patients with seizures to licensing authorities. Approximately 26% reported patients with dementia and 4–8% reported patients for stroke or other neurological disorders, respectively.

Physicians may also be cautious in reporting out of concern about violating their legal and ethical obligation to protect the privacy of communications and information about a patient's condition that inure to the physician–patient relationship (Galski et al., 2000; Pierce, 1993). Such obligation is reflected in the Hippocratic oath, medical ethics of the American Medical Association and common law (Hague v Williams, 37 NJ 328, 1962; AMA, 1971).

Physicians are, in fact, compelled to breach a patient's confidentiality and reveal "confidences entrusted in the course of medical attendance or deficiencies (they) may observe ..." relative to driving safety in States with mandatory reporting laws. Such a breach may be eased by the fact that a patient does not have an "absolute right but rather ... possesses a limited right against such disclosure, subject to exceptions prompted by the supervening interest of society" as well as relative certainty that courts would never hold a physician liable in any way for following statutory requirements (AMA, 1971).

In States that encourage voluntary reporting but do not statutorily require reporting persons whose condition could affect driving safety, physicians are not as clearly protected by law and may be less willing to risk alienation of a patient, perhaps litigation, by breaching confidentiality if perchance a safe driver is incorrectly reported to authorities. In addition to jeopardizing patient–physician relationship, some reluctance may be increased by recent changes in legislation that protect an individual's confidential information, such as the Health Insurance Portability and Accountability Act of 1996 (HIPAA).

However, physicians who report out of concern for their patients and the public and act in accordance with standards of care are usually granted immunity from liability for providing opinions and recommendations to the licensing authorities. Even when this is not explicitly provided by law, courts generally find that physicians who exercise reasonable care in making these reports are immune from liability for their actions (Illinois Vehicle Code, m 625 ILCS 5/6-109; Minnesota Regulations 7410.2500, R 7410.2600; Nevada Administrative Code, Chapter 483, Section 330; New Jersey Statutes 39:3 10.5; Vermont Code, Regulations 14-050-040; Washington Administrative Code 308-104-014). Nevertheless, physicians may expect damage to the physician–patient relationship by reporting any medical information to authorities that patients can perceive as a threat to licensure.

LICENSING AUTHORITY ACTION

Depending on the threat to the public safety posed by a driver and the need for balancing duties owed to drivers and society, licensing authorities are charged with issuance, suspension, revocation and, in most States, restriction of a person's license to drive. In cases involving medical issues, the commissioner, or director, of the licensing authority may obtain assistance from medical advisory boards, or panels, in an effort to give fair consideration to an applicant for licensure.

Medical advisory boards, established pursuant to authority of the licensing agency, are usually comprised of a select number of physicians from designated specialties (e.g., neurology or neurological surgery, cardiovascular medicine, internal medicine, family practice, ophthalmology, psychiatry, orthopedics, gerontology, and rehabilitative medicine), other professionals in relevant fields (e.g., optometry, psychology), and several lay members (Code of Alabama, Section 32–6: 40–46; Code of Maine Statutes, Title 29-A, Chapter 11, Section 1258; New Jersey Statutes, Title 39:2 13-15; New York State Consolidated Laws, Vehicle and Traffic, Article 21-B, Section 540–545; Vermont Title 23, Chapter 9, Section 637). Members are appointed by the director of the licensing agency and serve for a specified period of time, typically 2–3 years terms, without compensation. Members are granted immunity from liability in any action or proceeding. Generally, boards have responsibilities including but not limited to evaluating individual cases that may come to its attention, advising the director on medical criteria related to safe operation of motor vehicles, and recommending procedures and guidelines for licensing persons with physical and/or mental impairments.

Notably, while most States are vague in descriptions of the advisory board's practices and procedures and rarely articulate standards for evaluating cases that come before the boards, Illinois highlights the responsibilities and duties of medical licensing boards. For example, applications for initial or renewal licensing are submitted for evaluation to the medical advisory board when questionable medical reports have been received by the licensing authority (Illinois Administrative Code 1030.16). An individual member of the medical advisory board is assigned to review the case based on required medical expertise; the board member reviewing the case is given broad discretion in asking for and reviewing the information that may be relevant to determination of licensure, including requirement for medical examinations. A preliminary determination is made by the reviewing board member and submitted to the chairperson of the advisory board who then makes a formal determination regarding the driver's fitness to safely operate a motor vehicle. When the licensing authority receives the determination of the medical advisory board, action is taken to issue, revoke or restrict licensure and the driver is notified of the decision by the director of the licensing agency.

Drivers have the opportunity to contest decisions of the licensing authority within specified timeframes and in accordance with regulatory requirements. In Illinois, a driver who challenges the determination of the licensing authority has the right to a case review by a panel of three members of the medical advisory board who are selected by the chairperson. The driver may submit additional information to the panel as part of the appeal.

Interestingly, licensing authorities have been charged with a failure to follow their own rules and protect society and there are an increasing number of cases in which decisions by the licensing authorities have been challenged by drivers and, in some case, by third parties (Ormond v Garrett, 8 NC App 662, 1970; First Insurance Company of Hawaii, Ltd. v International Harvester Company, 66 Haw 185, 1983; Peterson v State of Washington, 100 Wash 2d 421, 1983; White v State Department of Public Safety and Corrections, 664 So 2d 684, La, 1994; written denied 684 So 2d 927, La, 1995).

SUMMARY

In conclusion, this brief review illustrates current legal procedures in the evaluation of driving capacity, which apply to both medically and non-medically involved individuals. Most notable is the variability in these legal procedures from State to State. This fact creates a significant challenge for clinicians faced with the task of advising neurologically compromised individuals about driving capacity. Nonetheless, a number of conclusions can be drawn from this brief review.

• Driving is a complex task requiring the interaction of physical, cognitive, perceptual, and psychological skills and abilities; impairments in one or more of these areas have been related to compromises in driving safety and addressed in laws governing licensure in all States.

• Driving safety is primarily related to and defined by frequency of accidents; risk of accidents varies amongst persons within a diagnostic category and between groups with different medical conditions depending on the nature and severity of the condition, interactive effects of treatments and co-morbidities and other variables.

• Epilepsy has historically been the primary medical condition focused on by licensing and regulating agencies, physicians and drivers; however, there are many medical conditions and/or medical treatments with associated or consequent impairments that can actually or potentially affect ability to safely operate a motor vehicle and increase risk of crashes.

• Laws, statutes, and codes are written in every State identifying medical and other conditions that may need to be brought to the attention of licensing authorities; however, in these regulations, there is (1) no uniformity amongst States about which conditions may pose a threat to patients and/or society and, therefore, require scrutiny by the licensing authorities; (2) no consensual agreement about the need for mandatory as opposed to voluntary reporting by physicians, patients themselves and/or other parties; and (3) a lack of clarity about the exact procedures to follow in reporting to the licensing agency.

• Physicians are identified in all States as the legally responsible parties for evaluating fitness to drive in patients with various medical conditions and for reporting their findings and recommendations to authorities on a mandatory or voluntary basis; however, physicians are compromised in their efforts by (1) a lack of clarity in defining potentially conflicting duties to patients and society; (2) a lack of guidelines for determining reasonably foreseeable danger of drivers with various medical conditions; (3) an absence of standardized, cost-effective, and proven methods to evaluate and predict real-world driver safety; (4) a limited familiarity with statutes and regulations governing evaluation and reporting of patients with specific medical conditions; and (5) insufficient education, training and experience to deal with functional tasks, such as driving, including an awareness of the multi-determinants of driving and effects of impairments on actual performance.

• Licensing agencies in all States seek driving-related information from physicians, drivers, and others mainly for use in estimating a driver's probability of accidents due to an identified medical condition or treatment; however, there are no defined cutoffs for low, moderate or high probabilities of accidents and no operationalized criteria on which to base decisions about licensure.

• Medical advisory boards may influence decisions about an individual's person's fitness to drive and standards for driving in the community; however, the role of advisory boards, their procedures and criteria for approving, denying or delimiting a person's driving privilege are not consistently and clearly articulated in written statutes and regulations across States.

• Patients who have medical conditions and/or are undergoing treatments that may compromise safety to operate a motor vehicle may continue to drive with a potentially increased risk of crashes and may not consistently self-report to the State licensing agency, perhaps out of ignorance or disregard of statutory requirements.

REFERENCES

Aarsland, D., Anderson, K., Larsen, J. P., Lolk, A., Nielsen, H., & Kragh-Sorensen, P. (2001). Risk of dementia in Parkinson's disease. A community-based, prospective study. *Neurology*, *56*(6), 730–736.

Aldrich, M. S. (1989). Automobile accidents in patients with sleep disorders. *Sleep*, *12*(6), 487–494.

American Medical Association (1971). *Code of Ethics*. Chicago: AMA.

Antrim, J. M., & Engum, E. S. (1989). The driving dilemma and the law: Patients' striving for independence vs. public safety. *Cognit. Rehabil.* (March–April), 16–19.

Arizona Administrative Code, Regulations 17-4-522 A1.

Ball, K., Owsley, C., Sloane, M. E., Roenker, D. L., & Bruni, J. R. (1993). Visual attention problems as a predictor of vehicle crashes in older drivers. *Investig. Opthalmol. Vis. Sci.*, *34*, 3110–3123.

Bor, F. L. (1990). A physician's warning and a warning to physicians. *NJ Rehabil.* (March), 20–22.

Calwell v Hassan, 925 P.2d 422 (Kan 1996).

Code of Alabama, Section 32-6: 40-46.

Code of Maine Regulations 29–250, Chapter 3, Section 2C-2D.

Code of Maine Statutes, Title 29-A, Chapter 11, Section 1258.

Code of Maryland Regulations 11.17.03.04.

Council on Ethical and Judicial Affairs (CEJA), American Medical Association. (1999). Report 4-A-99: Impaired drivers and their physicians.

Crancer, A., & McMurray, L. (1968). Accident and violation rates of Washington's medically restricted drivers. *J. Am. Med. Assoc.*, *205*, 272–276.

Crancer, A., & O'Neall, P. A. (1970). A record analysis of Washington drivers with license restrictions for heart disease. *Northwest Med.*, *69*, 409–416.

DC Municipal Regulations, Title 18, Sec 106.

DMV v Granziel, 236 NJ Super 191. Appellate Division, 1989.

Duvall v Goldin, 362 NW2d 275 (Mich Ct App 1984).

Evans, D. W., & Ginsburg, A. P. (1985). Contrast sensitivity predicts age-related differences in highway sign discriminability. *Hum. Factors*, *27*, 637–642.

Federal Rules of Evidence, Article VII, Rules 702–703.

First Insurance Company of Hawaii, Ltd. v International Harvester Company, 66 Haw 185, 1983.

Fitten, L. J. (1997). The demented driver: The doctor's dilemma. *Alzheimer Dis. Assoc. Disord.*(Suppl. 11), 1:57–:1:61.

Freese v Lemmon, 210 NW 2nd 576, Iowa, 1973.

Friedland, R. P., Koss, E., Kumar, A., Gaine, S., Metzler, D., Haxby, J. V., & Moore, A. (1988). Motor vehicle crashes in dementia of the Alzheimer type. *Ann. Neurol., 24*(6), 782–786.

Frier, B., Matthews, D. M., Steel, J. M., & Duncan, L. J. (1980). Driving and insulin-dependent diabetes. *Lancet, 1*(8180), 1232–1234.

Gallo, J. J., Rebok, G. W., & Lesikar, S. E. (1999). The driving habits of adults aged 60 years and older. *J. Am. Geriatr. Soc., 47*(3), 335–341.

Galski, T., Bruno, R. L., & Ehle, H. T. (1992). Driving after cerebral damage: A model with implications for evaluation. *Am. J. Occup. Ther., 46*, 324–332.

Galski, T., Ehle, H. T., & Bruno, R. L. (1993). Prediction of behind-the-wheel driving in patients with cerebral brain damage: A discriminant function analysis. *Am. J. Occup. Ther., 47*(5), 391–396.

Galski, T., Ehle, H. T., McDonald, M. A., & Mackevich, J. (2000). Evaluating fitness to drive after cerebral injury: Basic issues and recommendations for medical and legal communities. *J. Head Trauma Rehabil., 15*(3), 895–908.

Gooden v Tips, 651 SW 2d 364, Tex App Tyler, 1983.

Gurgold, G. D., & Harden, D. H. (1978). Assessing the driving potential of the handicapped. *Am. J. Occup. Ther., 32*, 41–46.

Hague v Williams, 37 NJ 328, 1962.

Hansotia, P., & Broste, S. K. (1991). The effect of epilepsy or diabetes mellitus on the risk of automobile accidents. *New Eng. J. Med., 32*(1), 22–26.

Hemmelgarn, B., Suissa, S., Huang, A., Boivin, J. F., & Pinard, G. (1997). Benzodiazepine use and the risk of motor vehicle crash in the elderly. *J. Am. Med. Assoc., 278*(1), 27–31.

Hopewell, C. A., & van Zomeren, A. H. (1990). Neuropsychological aspects of motor vehicle operations. In: D. E. Tupper, & K. Ciccerone (Eds.), *The Neuropsychology of Everyday Life: Assessment and Basic Competencies,* (pp. 72–90). Norwell, MA: Kluwer Academic Publishers.

Illinois Administrative Code 1030.16.

Illinois Vehicle Code, m 625 ILCS 5/6-109.

Jacobs, S. (1978). Reporting the handicapped driver. *Arch. Phys. Med. Rehabil., 59*, 387–390.

Kakaiya, R., Tisovec, R., & Fulkerson, P. (2000). Evaluation of fitness to drive. The physician's role in assessing elderly or demented patients. *Postgrad. Med. J., 107*(3), 229–236.

Kansas Administrative Regulations 92-52-11.

King, D., Benbow, S. J., & Barrett, J. A. (1992). The law and medical fitness to drive – A study of doctors' knowledge. *Postgrad. Med. J., 68*(802), 624–628.

Laberge-Nadeau, C., Dionne, G., Ekoe, J. M., Hamet, P., Desjardins, D., Messier, S., & Maag, U. (2000). Impact of diabetes on crash risks of truck-permit holders and commercial drivers. *Diabetes Care, 23*(5), 612–617.

Malinowski, M., & Petrucelli, E. (1997). Update of medical review practices and procedures in US and Canadian Driver License Program. Federal Highway Administration, Washington, DC (DT FH61-95-P-01200).

Masa, J. F., Rubio, M., & Findley, L. J. (2000). Habitually sleepy drivers have a high frequency of automobile crashes associated with respiratory disorders during sleep. *Am. J. Respir. Crit. Care Med., 162*(4 Pt 1), 1407–1412.

Mclachlan, R. S. (1997). Medical conditions and driving: Legal requirements and approach of neurologists. *Medical Law, 16*(2), 269–275.

Michigan Administrative Code, Regulations 257.851.

Minnesota Regulations 7410.2500, R 7410.2600.

Naidu v Laird, 539 A 2nd 1064, Del Sup, 1988.

Nevada Administrative Code Chapter 483, Sec 330.

New Jersey Administrative Code 13:19-4.1-5.10.

New Jersey Statutes, Motor Vehicles and Traffic, Title 39:3 10.5.

New Jersey Statutes, Motor Vehicles and Traffic, Title 39:2 13–15.

New York Comprehensive Codes, Rules and Regulations. Title 15, Section 9.1–9.3.

New York State Consolidated Laws, Vehicles and Traffic, Article 21-B, Section 540–545.

Ormond v Garrett, 8 N.C. App 662, 1970.

Owsley, C., Ball, K., Sloane, M., Roenker, D., & Bruni, J. (1991). Visual/cognitive correlates of vehicle accidents in older drivers. *Psychol. Aging, 6,* 403–415.

Peterson v State of Washington, 100 Wash 2d 421, 1983.

Pidikiti, R. D., & Novack, T. A. (1991). The disabled driver: An unmet challenge. *Arch. Phys. Med. Rehabil., 72*(2), 109–111.

Pierce, S. (1978). Legal considerations for a driver rehabilitation program. *Phys. Disabil. (Special Issue on Driver Rehabilitation), 16*(1), 1–4.

Pierce, S. (1993). Legal considerations for a driver rehabilitation program. Special Interest Section Newsletter. *AOTA, 72,* 109–111.

Popkin, C.L., & Waller, P.F. (1988). Epilepsy and driving in North Carolina: An exploratory study. In: *32nd Annual Proceedings of the Association for the Advancement of Automotive Medicine* (pp. 347–358). Des Plaines, IL.

Reuben, D. B., Silliman, R. A., & Traines, M. (1998). The aging driver: Medicine, policy and ethics. *JAGS, 36,* 1135–1142.

Schultheis, M. T., Garay, E., & DeLuca, J. (2001). The influence of cognitive impairment on driving performance in multiple sclerosis. *Neurology, 56*(8), 1089–1094.

Sivak, M., Olson, P. L., Kewman, D. G., Won, H., & Henson, D. L. (1981). Driving and perceptual/cognitive skills: Behavioral consequences of brain damage. *Arch. Phys. Med. Rehabil., 62,* 476–483.

State v Zoppi, 196 NJ Super 596, Law Division, 1984.

Tarasoff v Regents of University of California, 17 Cal 3d 425, Sup Ct, 1976.

Vermont Code, Regulations 14-050-040.

Vermont Title 23, Motor Vehicles, Chapter 9, Section 637.

Waller, J. A. (1965). Chronic medical conditions and traffic safety: A review of California Experience. *New Eng. J. Med., 273,* 1413–11420.

Waller, J. A. (1967). Cardiovascular disease, ageing, and traffic accidents. *J. Chron. Dis., 20,* 615–620.

Waller, J., & Goo, J. T. (1969). Highway crash and citation patterns and chronic medical conditions. *J. Saf. Res., 1,* 13–27.

Washington Administrative Code 308-104-014.

White v State Department of Public Safety and Corrections, 664 So 2d 684, La, 1994; written denied 684 So 2d 927, La, 1995.

Wilschinsky v Medina, 775P.2d 713 (NM 1989).

11

FINAL THOUGHTS AND FUTURE DIRECTIONS

MARIA T. SCHULTHEIS

While much work has been completed in examining driving performance in a variety of clinical populations, there remains much work to be done. Studies to date compile a large literature, much of which has been presented in the previous chapters. While our goal was to present a comprehensive review, we recognize that the information is not all-inclusive and other work in the field of driving contributes greatly to our overall understanding of driving after a neurological compromise. For example, research with older and younger drivers, studies including other clinical populations (e.g. ADHD, psychiatric) and transportation research on the development and evaluation of driving tools. Yet, the knowledge that has been acquired through the various studies presented can allow us to draw some conclusions about what we know and what challenges remain in the field of clinical driving assessment. The goal of this chapter is to highlight these findings by summarizing the lessons learned and providing a discussion about challenges that remain to be addressed.

SECTION I: LESSONS LEARNED

A MULTI-LEVEL COMPREHENSIVE DRIVING ASSESSMENT IS RECOMMENDED FOR DETERMINING DRIVING CAPACITY

The results of studies from various clinical populations have all provided evidence that driving is a complex task, and subsequently, the assessment of driving capacity after neurological compromise is an equally complex task. As outlined in the previous chapters, driving capacity can be affected by a variety of impairments, including physical, sensory, cognitive, emotional, and behavioral challenges. And despite the fact, that in some diagnoses or clinical groups, specific factors may be more prominent, this does not preclude the need for a comprehensive assessment of all the domains.

As early as 1990, Katz et al., identified the importance of a comprehensive driving assessment and while today, the current gold standard for determining fitness to drive is the behind-the-wheel (BTW) evaluation (described in Chapter 1), many clinicians charged with the responsibility of evaluating driving capacity support the notion of providing a comprehensive evaluation. In particular, this would include assessment by trained clinicians in specific domains. For example, driving specialist, who often are trained in occupation therapy, will commonly refer individuals to an ophthalmologist to provide a thorough visual examination. By the same token, if can be argued that a clinical neuropsychologist should be engaged to provide a cognitive evaluation and a physician can provide a comprehensive medical examination.

In sum, the findings from the research studies would endorse a multi-level driving assessment that includes the following components: medical, visual, cognitive, driving evaluation, and education. Specifically, at the most basic level, evaluation of basic visual and medical status would be necessary to establish that the individual meets minimum physical and sensory criteria for operating a motor vehicle. In addition, a comprehensive medical examination can help identify any possible conflicts with medications or secondary medical issues that may warrant monitoring or re-evaluation of driving capacity. In addition, a comprehensive cognitive assessment should be completed to identify any specific deficits in cognitive domains relevant to driving. The next level should include a comprehensive driving evaluation including both off- and on-road evaluations of driving performance. If available, driving simulation can be used to compliment the driving assessment, by allowing simulated assessment of driving in challenging scenarios. Finally, a component that is not commonly considered is education. This last component should not only provide an overview of areas of concern, but also discussion of alternate transportation (if necessary) and potential areas that may require re-evaluation or training.

THE INFLUENCE OF COGNITIVE IMPAIRMENT ON DRIVING HAS BEEN IDENTIFIED IN A VARIETY OF CLINICAL POPULATIONS

Although many may view driving as a physically demanding task (e.g., turning steering wheel, pushing pedals), the impact of cognitive functioning on driving skills and abilities is one of the most robust finding in the clinical driving literature. Findings from several neurological populations demonstrate that decline in cognition negatively impacts performance on driving-related measures. Early work demonstrated this relationship in populations with moderate to severe cognitive impairments, such as traumatic brain injury (van Zomeren et al., 1987; Galski et al., 1993), stroke (Mazer et al., 1998; Akinwuntan et al., 2006), and dementia (Cox et al., 1998). More recently research has examined this relationship among populations that demonstrate milder levels of cognitive compromise, such as attention-deficit hyperactivity disorder (ADHD) (Woodward et al., 2000; Barkley et al., 2002), human immunodeficiency virus (HIV) (Marcotte et al., 2004), and multiple sclerosis (MS) (Schultheis et al., 2001, 2002). The combined results of these studies offer evidence that the relationship between cognition and driving can be seen across the broad spectrum of cognitive impairment. Specifically, the cognitive domains most consistently reported include: attention, information processing speed, working memory, visuo-spatial, and visual perceptual skills, underscoring their important contribution to driving performance.

OTHER FACTORS CAN INFLUENCE DRIVING CAPACITY

In addition to physical and cognitive factors, evidence across the various studies indicates that factors that are secondary or independent of the primary diagnosis can also influence driving performance. Among these, quite a bit has been discussed about the impact of medications, including studies on medications commonly used to treat depression and anxiety (Wingen et al., 2005), conditions commonly seen among individuals with neurological compromise. Given the great variability in the types of pharmacological interventions that are available, not only must clinicians consider the impact of individual medications, but also the potential for issues of poly-pharmacology. In addition, while some medications types such as sedatives, may have negative effects on driving performance, other types, such as those increasing attention and concentration may prove beneficial (at least in specific clinical diagnosis, e.g., ADHD). Regardless, findings from the handful of studies that have explored this topic indicate the need for clinicians to both inquire and educate individuals about the potential impact of medication on driving performance (Summers, 2004).

Another important factor to consider in the evaluation of driving capacity is the potential impact of concomitant disorders. For example, sleep disorders can have significant effects on an individuals' ability to operate a motor vehicle (Volna & Sonka, 2006). Some specific types of sleep disorders such a narcolepsy may preclude an individual from driving; however, other more subtle disturbances in sleep can also have a negative effect and have been shown to have a higher incidence following TBI (Mahmood et al., 2004). Other systemic disorders may also have an influence on an individual's cognitive and physical/sensory abilities which may impact driving capacity, for example, hypertension, diabetes, and disturbances in vision (e.g., glaucoma).

While the role of emotions on driving performance may be examined clinically in relation to issues of anxiety or depression, a significant amount of research has been reported in studies of non-clinical drivers. For example, findings from a recent study indicate that individuals who drive while reporting feelings of anger are more likely to drive faster and exceed speed limits (Mesken et al., 2007) and fear has been correlated with higher number of driving errors (Taylor et al., 2007). Along this line, studies have focused on personality factors or individual characteristics that may increase risk for unsafe driving. For example, one recent longitudinal study that followed a cohort of 1,037 young adults, found that among male drivers aggression, traditionalism, and alienation were the personality scales most frequently associated with risky driving behavior and crash risk (Gulliver & Begg, 2007). Impulsive and risk taking behaviors have also been a main focus of this line of research.

A final factor to consider in evaluating driving capacity includes the overall social environment or realm of the individual. Among this, one can consider issues such as dependence on driving, the influence of significant others, and issues of substance abuse. In fact, recent research has demonstrated that an individual's perceived barriers to driving is one of the strongest predictors of return to driving after neurological compromise (e.g., brain injury) (Rapport et al., 2006). Subsequently, among clinical populations where limitation in self-awareness or limited awareness of deficit (e.g., dementia) may arise, clinicians are encouraged to work not only with the individual but with significant others and/or family members to more accurately assess readiness to drive.

In sum, while much of the clinical literature has focused on identifying the cognitive demands of driving and predicting driving performance after neurological compromise, other factors warrant consideration. While research examining these other factors has been mainly limited to non-clinical samples, the findings have relevant implications for clinical populations. The need for incorporating assessment of factors such as medication, emotionality, personality, and social influences further supports the recommendation for comprehensive, multi-level assessment of driving. In addition, the variability of factors to consider underscores the benefit of having experts in the specific field conduct the specific area of evaluation (e.g., medication by physician, cognition by neuropsychologist, social/emotional by psychologist), these experts can assess and address these contributing factors both at an individual level but also as a component to the more holistic contribution to driving capacity.

LEGAL ISSUES AND REGULATIONS ARE AN IMPORTANT COMPONENT OF DRIVING ASSESSMENT

There is only one consensus in regard to legal issues related to driving assessment, and that is that great variability exists. Indeed, due to the lack of federal regulations, licensure and reporting procedures vary greatly from state to state, making it the clinician's responsibility to be aware of what is expected in cases where driving capacity is in question.

Those clinicians faced with the direct task of assessing driving and those faced with the task of referring for a driving assessment are encouraged to familiarize themselves with state laws regarding: (1) mandate to report, (2) availability of anonymous reporting, and (3) reporting procedures. In addition, individuals working within settings where driving issues may arise frequently (e.g., medical and rehabilitation institutions) are encouraged to identify a plan of action for managing questions about driving capacity.

Legally, clinicians should familiarize themselves with the specific laws of their practicing state. For example, not all states have mandatory reporting laws, some are permissive. In addition, each state has its own definition of what is considered impairment to driving. Some may list specific disorders, such as seizure activity, while other states may have more generic descriptions of what observations would require reporting. Clinicians should also note that some states carry monetary fines for failure to report, and in other states (e.g., Pennsylvania) clinicians can be found negligent to report a driver who is later involved in an accident. A summary chart of some key aspects of driving regulations in the 50 states is provided in Appendix A; however, clinician are encouraged to directly contact the motor vehicle agency of their state.

Regardless of the legal responsibilities, for physician and other clinicians, there is also the ethical responsibility to report an individual who may not be able to drive safely. As such, an a priori plan of action is often recommended and should include at minimum the following aspects:

a. Know the law
b. Identify pathway for referral (e.g., driver center information)
c. Be alert to potential driving impairments
d. Inquire about driving habits
e. Intervene and educate individuals of potential driving challenges
f. Identify alternative transportation options.

EDUCATION AND FOLLOW-UP ARE IMPORTANT COMPONENTS OF DRIVING ASSESSMENT

Too often, when issues of driving capacity arise, the focus is on determining whether an individual can or cannot continue to drive at that point in time. What is commonly lost, are consideration for issues such as driver training and the potential need for follow-up or re-assessment. In fact, in a recent survey of driving evaluation practices in both the United States and Canada, clinicians reported that the majority of their time was allocated to assessment and not retraining (Korner-Bitensky et al., 2006).

This fact is further exemplified in a brief review of the clinical driving literature, which although extensive, only includes a small percentage of studies that have examined driver retraining or driver education. In terms of driver retraining, some researchers have examined the use of computerized tasks to improve aspects of visual attention and reaction time (Mazer et al., 2003). Others have employed the use of driving simulators to improve driving performance

(Akinwuntan et al., 2005). In general, the findings from this handful of studies are inconclusive, and additional work is needed to more accurately define the best driver retraining methodology for these neurologically compromised groups. However, some helpful information can be derived from a recent review of driver training among older drivers. Specifically, these researchers conducted a systematic and critical appraisal of the existing evidence for the effectiveness of driver retraining procedures for older adults. Their findings indicated that there was little support for the effectiveness for models focusing on physical retraining or visual perception retraining (Kua et al., 2007). By contrast moderate evidence was found for education interventions in improving driving awareness and driving behavior, but did not reduce crashes among older drivers (Kua et al., 2007). Subsequently, at minimum clinicians are encouraged to educate individuals about potential driving difficulties and factors that may increase driving difficulties, ask questions about driving behaviors and engage in discussion about driving with their patients.

A second component that is commonly not addressed as part of the driving assessment is the concept of re-assessment or follow-up. In particular, most individuals report only receiving one driver evaluation following their injury or diagnosis. Yet, many individuals may benefit from a follow-up and re-evaluation after some period of time. First, it is important to consider the progressive nature of some disorders, such as dementia or MS. In fact, the progressive nature of MS is clinically well-established and recent research findings have demonstrated a relationship between cognitive impairment in MS and driving performance (Schultheis et al., 2001); yet, little to no research exists examining how this relationship changes over the course of the disease. Similarly, in individual diagnosed with dementia; the prognosis is often an increase in impairments with resulting loss of capacity to perform everyday activities. Yet, there are no clear guidelines for clinicians to recommend initial and follow-up evaluations of driving capacity as the dementia progresses. In addition to the progressive nature of disorders, re-assessment may also be valuable among individuals aging with a neurological compromise (e.g., aging with TBI). Specifically, it has been argued that these individuals may be at a higher risk for driving difficulties due to cognitive and behavioral impairments that may result from the co-existing disorders (Brenner et al., 2008).

In sum, clinicians are encouraged to view the driving assessment, not as a "one time" evaluation, but rather to consider driving performance within the scope of the individual's day-to-day activities. This may result in identification of opportunities for retraining skills relevant to driving, as well as provide early identification of potential changes in the individual that may warrant a re-evaluation.

SECTION II: CHALLENGES THAT REMAIN

As with any growing field of research, it is not uncommon to note that while much has been learned from previous work, there are several overarching areas that continue to require additional research to improve our ability to understand and adequately assess driving performance after neurological compromise.

IDENTIFICATION OF ADEQUATE CRITERION FOR THE DETERMINATION OF FITNESS TO DRIVE

Although the task of defining driving performance would appear to be straightforward, it is in actuality a challenge to attempt to quantify successful driving behavior. Defining a standard and accepted criterion of driving performance has been a long-standing challenge within the driving research community. Subsequently, there is great variability in what defines successful driving, resulting in a lack of consensus of what is acceptable or non-acceptable behavior.

At present, the most commonly used criterion is the pass versus fail performance on an "on-road" or "behind-the-wheel" driver evaluation. Indeed, the majority of the clinical research studies conducted with drivers with neurological compromise rely on this measure to define driving performance (Galski et al., 1990; Fox et al., 1998; Mazer et al., 1998). However, there are several limitations that reduce the validity of this measure as a criterion for driving performance. First, the great majority of on-road assessments are based on subjective observations of driving performance that is commonly conducted within a 1-hour time frame (in many cases less), on a route that is selected by the evaluator. As a result, there is a lack of standardization in procedures for an on-road assessment and indeed, no two are exactly alike. Coupled with the subjective nature of the evaluation, it is not surprising that great variability exist in what can be defined as "pass" or fail" performance. Second, it is important to consider that the "on-road" represents only a snapshot of the person's driving capacity. Due to the time limits and also the safety considerations, this demonstration of driving does not offer examples of how individuals will perform under more challenging conditions and/or what their performance would be during routine driving (i.e., not under evaluation). Taken together, the use of the pass versus fail performance on an on-road driver evaluation significantly limits the ability to evaluate what can be defined as "real-world driving". In fact, a common criticism of studies that rely solely on this measure is that on-road performance does not represent what the individual will do behind the wheel once they have regained their driving privileges. Although there is little argument that the "on-road" is an important component of the assessment of driving capacity (as part of a multi-level evaluation), its role as a criterion for driving capacity is limited at best.

A second measure commonly used to define driving performance is the frequency of motor vehicle accidents and/or violations. Many have argued that this measure allows for a better representation of what individual's do in "everyday driving". Indeed, this criterion can provide a more objective measurement of driving performance, in particular when reports from the department of motor vehicle (DMV) are used as the source of documentation. However, it is not without flaw. One of the major limitations of this measure is the low frequency of actual documented accidents or violations. This is further confounded by the fact that most studies have only examined frequency of motor vehicle incidents for short term (e.g., 6 months) and not long term (greater than 1 year) follow-up. Furthermore, specific information about the incident is often difficult to obtain, as most DMV reports do not offer specific details about the nature of the incident (e.g., who is at fault). Some researchers have relied on self-report to obtain information about accidents and driving violations; however, the reliability of this information is often questioned.

In sum, the lack of an accepted criterion for quantifying driving performance is a significant limitation in the existing literature of driving research among clinical populations. A lack of consensus on a criterion, limits the interpretability of the numerous studies and limits the opportunity to merge the knowledge that has been gained across the studies. One potential solution is the use of multiple driving performance measures within a study (e.g., on-road and DMV reports). Another is to increase the length of follow-up time to capture more realistic representation of driving behaviors. Research that aims to standardize how we measure driving and improves the objective measurement of driving behaviors would significantly improve our ability to integrate findings from across the various clinical populations. Until this time, the reported findings are limited to a particular study or sample and minimize the ability to advance the science.

INCORPORATING NEW TECHNOLOGIES TO THE ASSESSMENT OF DRIVING

The use of new technologies has provided numerous advances in various aspects of science. Not surprisingly, in the field of driving research, technology can also help address many of the limitations of current clinical driving assessment methods. One particular technology is the use of simulation or the development of driving simulators. The benefits of a driving simulators have been described by previous researchers and are summarized in Table 11.1 (adapted from Schultheis & Mourant, 2001).

Researchers from Canada were one of the first to introduced a virtual reality (VR)-based driving simulator (VRDS) for clinical assessment, the DriVR (Liu et al., 1999; Wald et al., 2000; Wald & Liu, 2001). The DriVR system is a PC-based interactive driving simulator that presents a variety of driving scenarios, calculates performance measures, and generates a profile of driving skills and behaviors deemed relevant to driving. Several studies have been conducted using the DriVR to establish its validity, it remains a promising, and now commercially available (www.driVR.com) research tool.

In the United States, research by Schultheis et al., has focused on the development of a clinically accessible VRDS. Specifically, this research is not focused on the use of a high-end simulator that is costly and requires dedicated space and personnel. Rather, this research focuses on a driving simulator that requires low-end, affordable technology (e.g., off-the-shelf).

TABLE 11.1 Comparison of VR Driving Assessment to Traditional Driving Assessment Protocols.

Current driving assessment protocols	Limitations	How VRDS addresses limitations
Cognitive tests	• Assess only individualized, not complex behaviors and skills • Questionable ecological validity	• Allow assessment of "complex" behaviors, such as driving • Allows assessment of driving skills in "real-life" situations
Computerized tasks	• Simplified graphics • Limited user interaction	• Interactive, detailed, "real-life" graphics • Maximum user interaction
Traditional driving simulators	• Variability in level of interaction • Financially inaccessible	• Submersive effect allows higher level of interaction • Increased advances in technology allow for a financially achievable system
Clinical BTW evaluations	• Based on subjective observations • Limited driving scenarios due to safety • Non-standardized procedures	• Allows for objective recording of all driving measures and behaviors • Easily modifiable environment allows assessment under various conditions • Controlled environment allows for safe evaluation of driving in complex and challenging situations • Allows for standardized assessment

While recent trends in driving research have focused on the identification of screening tools for the prediction of driver involvement (e.g., brief physiological and/or cognitive measurements) these researchers have built a VRDS designed to compliment current clinical driving assessment methods. Unlike the brief screening tasks that have been the focus of driving research which can be more convenient from a driver rehabilitation perspective, the VRDS assesses driving as a complex behavior that requires the integration of multiple cognitive domains. Additionally, the use of a driving simulator can provide more detailed information and allows specific and objective driving performance measures which can help to inform driver assessment feedback and guide driver retraining. Finally, VRDS has a greater degree of face validity than the current assessment tools and clinically, this can be a significant factor in acceptance of impaired performance among individuals.

The VRDS allows the user to "drive through" a specified route with a variety of driving zones (e.g., highway, residential, commercial, school). The virtual route takes approximately 30 minutes to administer and offers the option to present a variety of "challenging" driving situations. For example, a pedestrian suddenly crossing the street or speeding vehicles entering the highway. The VRDS automatically records four primary measures of driving behavior while the individual is driving through the route, these includes speed of the vehicle, lane position, head turning position, and distance from target object (i.e., stop signs, traffic lights). These preliminary driving behaviors were selected based on prior VR programming experience (Mourant & Ge, 1999; Mourant et al., 2001) and clinical experience. Additional driving performance measures can be calculated from combinations of the four primary output measures. To date, research with the VRDS has included both healthy, normal drivers and individuals with neurological compromise (i.e., stroke, brain injury).

Using the VRDS, Schultheis et al. demonstrated the use of VRDS to measure more specific behaviors of driving, such as driving behaviors for managing a stop sign intersection. Given the high risk associated with stop sign management among normal drivers, we examined specific measures of driving performance related to stop sign intersections among 15 drivers with acquired brain injury and compared them to 9 healthy controls (Schultheis et al., 2006). Comparison of these measures found a pattern of improved performance with repeated exposure. As expected both groups demonstrated atypical performance at initiation (Stop Sign 1). This was due to unfamiliarity with the VRDS and the virtual environment and a lack of depth and perceptual accommodation. Interestingly, while both groups showed learning patterns across the three stop sign intersections, the observed patterns were different between the two groups. While between-group differences were not anticipated, the findings indicate some differences in performance with disability (with the ABI group showing greater difficulties). This is despite the fact that both groups were matched on driving experience, and that the ABI group included only drivers who had regained driving privileges.

A second auxiliary benefit of using a VRDS is the face validity it offers. Specifically, because VR driving so closely resembles real-life driving, it is often well-received by patients, family members, and clinicians. In fact, in a recent study we attempted to quantify the overall user ratings regarding comfort and reception of the VRDS among individuals with stroke, brain injury, and healthy controls (Schultheis et al., 2007). Our results indicated that overall all three groups gave favorable ratings to the use of the VRDS, with healthy control providing the highest ratings, followed by brain injury users and stroke users.

Although promising, research in the development of driving simulators for clinical assessment of driving capacity is still in the early stages and additional work will be needed to validate the use of this technology as a new clinical tool. Most importantly, work is still needed to establish the validity of simulation performance as a measure of "real-world" driving performance. Although the potential for additional benefits of driving simulation are often discussed, more work is also need to examine potential negative aspects of using this technology. In particular, consideration of the impact of this technology on clinical populations is warranted.

For example, research using simulation has demonstrated that individuals can experience "simulation sickness," a condition similar to motion sickness, which can create feelings of discomfort, nausea, and dizziness. Evaluation of the incident of simulation sickness would be necessary prior to the use of a driving simulator with clinical populations. Another consideration is the impact of "familiarity with technology." Although many individuals today are exposed early to technologies, older adults may not have a similar experience and subsequently may not be comfortable in the use of such driving simulators. Discomfort with the technology could subsequently confound the driving performance that is observed during simulated drives, and could result in inaccurate representation of an individual's capacity (see Simone et al., 2006).

In sum, one technology that has been extensively examined in driving research is the use of driving simulators. And while, these simulators may serve to address the various limitations that are present in the current clinical driving assessment methods, further research is needed to establish the clinical utility and the validity of driving performance based on simulation.

INCORPORATING A TRANSDISCIPLINARY APPROACH IN DRIVING ASSESSMENT

In our fast-paced society driving is a privilege that represents independence and freedom to many individuals. As a result information and knowledge about driving is important at both the societal level, as well as the individual level. While, we have attempted to summarize the research and findings from studies that have focused on examining driving among individuals with neurological compromise, the information presented is miniscule compared to the vast literature that is compiled within the field of transportation research. What is remarkable and discouraging is the clear separation between these two bodies of research that are examining the same concept.

Transportation research has a long history, which includes research from established fields such as the military, the automobile industry, and highway and transportation agencies. The individuals working in this field, typically come from a variety of backgrounds, and can include expertise in human factors, cognitive psychology, various types of engineering (e.g., mechanical, usability), and computer science. Despite the clear differences in the individuals involved in transportation research, the similarities are in the research that is conducted by this group. For example, transportation research includes work examining human driving errors, driver distraction, driver fatigue, and investigating the cognitive workload of driving task. These studies examine differences in novice versus experienced drivers, age-related driving errors, and the relationship between personality and driving. While this represents only a small list of topics studied and published within the area of transportation research, the overlap with the interests of clinical research on driving is obvious.

Unlike, clinical driving research, the use of technologies in transportation research is not a novel approach but rather an accepted methodology. For example, the use of instrumented vehicles is well-established and has been used to monitor visual search behaviors during driving (Recarte & Nunes, 2000), examine the relationship between personality and driving styles (Boyce & Geller, 2002), examine differences in driving experience between novice and experienced drivers (Witman et al., 1998) and to evaluate driver fatigue (Veeraraghavan & Papaniklopoulos, 2001). More recently, there have been a few studies that have applied video-based observation to study driving of at-risk older drivers (Crowe et al., 2001). Similarly, a large body of work exists that has relied on driving simulation for defining aspects of human driving performance. The findings from these studies have served to establish a better understanding of driving behavior, and have contributed to the identification of factors that have a direct impact on improving the safety of our roads. For example, research using driving simulation has helped to identify the most frequent causes of automobile collisions (Cox et al., 1999; Fiorentino et al., 1997), delineate the various contributors to human driving error (Ivancic & Hesketh, 2000), identify factors that have the most negative impact on driving performance (Menefee et al., 2004) and contributed to the development of new devices that can assist drivers and reduce the risk of collision (Ben-Yaacov et al., 2002). More recent studies have used simulators to understand driver attention and examine the impact of devices (e.g., cellular phones) on driving ability (Greenberg et al., 2003).

To date, much of the transportation research has focused on normal driving performance, and subsequently the studies have provided useful information into identifying what variables most accurately reflect driving performance in healthy adult drivers. However, examination into whether these specific measures of driving performance are also meaningful in clinical populations, has yet to be explored. Other questions include whether performance is the same or whether there are other salient driving performance measures that should be considered when neurological compromise is present.

In many ways, in comparison to transportation research the clinical driving research literature may appear trivial. But in fact, clinical research can bring several unique aspects to transportation research. For example, research with clinical populations can help provide an understanding of the broad spectrum of human behaviors versus only examining "normal" drivers. Clinical research also offers an opportunity for long-term follow-up to examine how driving behaviors may change over time and with changes to the individual, unlike the shorter term focus more commonly used in transportation research.

In sum, one area of necessary growth to help expand the science of driving is integration of transdisciplinary knowledge. In essence, without this collaboration, the information gathered will be limited and will not allow true investigation of more complex questions about driving after neurological compromise. In particular, the clinical research may lack the necessary information for the development of clinically relevant tools that can enhance clinical decision making.

CONCLUSION

The main objective of this book was to provide a reference for clinicians that included a clear description of current clinical methods for assessing driving capacity following neurological compromise and an overview of the existing body of research and relevant issues related to the assessment of driving following neurological compromise. While an all-inclusive review was beyond the scope of this book, the goal was to bring to light the key issues for clinicians to be able to make practical everyday decisions about driving.

REFERENCES

Akinwuntan, A. E., De Weedt, W., Feys, H., Pauwels, J., Baten, G., Arno, P., & Kiekens, C. (2005). Effect of simulator training on driving after stroke: A randomized controlled trial. *Neurology*, *65*(6), 843–850.

Akinwuntan, A. E., Feys, H., De Weerdt, W., Baten, G., Arno, P., & Kiekens, C. (2006). Prediction of driving after stroke: A prospective study. *Neurorehabil. Neural Repair*, *20*(3), 417–423.

Barkley, R. A., Murphy, K. R., Dupaul, G. J., & Bush, T. (2002). Driving in young adults with attention deficit hyperactivity disorder: Knowledge, performance, adverse outcomes, and the role of executive functioning. *J. Int. Neuropsychol. Soc.*, *8*, 655–672.

Ben-Yaacov, A., Maltz, M., & Shinar, D. (2002). Effects of an in-vehicle collision avoidance warning system on short and long-term driving performance. *J. Hum. Fact. Ergon. Soc.*, *44*(2), 335–342.

Brenner, L., Homaifer, B., & Schultheis, M. T. (2008). Driving, Aging and Traumatic Brain Injury: Integrating findings from the literature. *Rehabilitation Psychology*, *53*(1), 18–27.

Boyce, T. E., & Geller, E. S. (2002). An instrumented vehicle assessment of problem behavior and driving style: Do younger males take more risks? *Accid. Anal. Prev.*, *34*, 51–64.

Cox, D. J., Quillian, W. C., Thorndike, F. P., Kovatchev, B. P., & Hanna, G. (1998). Evaluating driving performance of outpatients with Alzheimer disease. *J. Am. Board Fam. Pract.*, *11*, 264–271.

Cox, D. J., Taylor, P., & Kovatchev, B. (1999). Driving simulation performance predicts future accidents among older drivers. *JAGS*, *47*(3), 381–382.

Crowe, A., Smyser, T., Raby, M., Bateman, K., & Rizzo, M. (2001). Visual attention and road-way landmark detection in at-risk older drivers. In: *Proceeding from "Driver Assessment, 2001"*. Aspen, Colorado.

Fiorentino, Dary D., & Zareh Parseghian (1997) "Time-to-collision: A sensitive measure of driver interaction with traffic in a simulated driving task," In: *Proceedings of the Human Factors and Ergonomics Society, 41st Annual Meeting* (pp. 1028–1031). Albuquerque, New Mexico.

Fox, G., Bowden, S., & Smith, D. (1998). On-road assessment of driving competence after brain impairment: Review of current practice and recommendations for standardized examination. *Arch. Phys. Med. Rehabil.*, *79*(10), 1288–1296.

Galski, T., Bruno, R. L., & Ehle, H. T. (1993). Prediction of behind-the-wheel driving performance in patients with cerebral brain damage: A discriminant function analysis. *Am. J. Occup. Ther.*, *47*, 391–396.

Galski, T., Ehle, H. T., & Bruno, R. L. (1990). An assessment of measures to predict the outcome of driving evaluations in patients with cerebral damage. *Am. J. Occup. Ther.*, *44*, 709–713.

Greenberg, J., Tijerina, L., Curry, R., Artz, B., Cathey, L., Kochhar, D. et al. (2003). Driver distraction evaluation with event detection paradigm. *Transportation Research Record: Journal of the Transportation Research Board*, *1843*, 1–8.

Gulliver, P., & Begg, D. (2007). Personality Factors as Predictors of Persistent Risky Driving Behavior and Crash Involvement among Young Adults. *Injury Prevention, 13*(6), 376–381.

Ivancic, K., & Hesketh, B. (2000). Learning from errors in a driving simulation: Effects on driving skill and self-confidence. *Ergonomics, 43*(12), 1966–1984.

Katz, R. T., Golden, R. S., Butter, J., Tepper, D., Rothke, S., Holmes, J., & Sahgal, V. (1990). Driving safety after brain damage: follow-up of twenty-two patients with matched controls. *Archives of Physical Medicine & Rehabilitation, 71*(2), 133–137.

Korner-Bitensky, N., Bitensky, J., Sofer, S., Man-Son-Hing, M., & Gelinas, I. (2006 Jul.–Aug.). Driving evaluation practices of clinicians working in the United States and Canada. *Am. J. Occup. Ther., 60*(4), 428–434.

Kua, A., Korner-Bitensky, N., Desrosiers, J., Man-Son-Hing, M., & Marshall, S. (2007). Older driver retraining: A systematic review of evidence of effectiveness. *J. Safety Res., 38*(1), 81–90. Epub 2007 Feb 14.

Liu, L., Miyazaki, M., & Watson, B. (1999). Norms and validity of the DriVR: A virtual reality driving assessment for persons with head injuries. *Cyberpsychology and Behavior, 2*(1), 53–67.

Mahmood, O., Rapport, L. J., Hanks, R. A., & Fichtenberg, N. L. (2004 Sep.–Oct.). Neuropsychological performance and sleep disturbance following traumatic brain injury. *J. Head Trauma Rehabil., 19*(5), 378–390.

Marcotte, T. D., Wolfson, T., Rosenthal, T. J., Heaton, R. K., Gonzalez, R., Ellis, R. J. et al. (2004). A multimodal assessment of driving performance in HIV infection. *Neurology, 63*, 1417–1422.

Mazer, B. L., Korner-Bitensky, N. A., & Sofer, S. (1998). Predicting ability to drive after stroke. *Arch. Phys. Med. Rehabil., 79*, 743–750.

Mazer, B. L., Sofer, S., Korner-Bitensky, N., Gelinas, I., Hanley, J., & Wood-Dauphinee, S. (2003 Apr.). Effectiveness of a visual attention retraining program on the driving performance of clients with stroke. *Arch. Phys. Med. Rehabil., 84*(4), 541–550.

Menefee, L. A., Frank, E. D., Crerand, C., Jalali, S., Park, J., Sanschagrin, K., & Besser, M. (2004). The effects of transdermal fentanyl on driving, cognitive performance, and balance in patients with chronic nonmalignant pain conditions. *Pain Med., 5*(1), 42–49.

Mesken, J., Hagenzieker, M. P., Rothengatter, T., & de Waard, D. (2007). Frequency, determinants, and consequences of different drivers' emotions: An on-the-road study using self-reports, (observed) behaviour, and physiology. *Transportation Research Part F: Traffic Psychology and Behaviour, 10*(6), 458–475.

Mourant, R. R., & Ge, Z. (1999). Measuring attentional demand in a virtual environment driving simulator. Proceedings of the 41st Annual Meeting of the Human Factors and Ergonomics Society, 1268–1272.

Mourant, R. R., Tsai, F-J., Al-Shihabi, T., & Jaeger, B. K. (2001). Measuring divided attention capacity among young and older drivers. *Transportation Research Record,* No. 1779, 40–45.

Rapport, L. J., Hanks, R. A., & Bryer, R. C. (2006 Jan.–Feb.). Barriers to driving and community integration after traumatic brain injury. *J. Head Trauma Rehabil., 21*(1), 34–44.

Recarte, M. A., & Nunes, L. M. (2000). Effects of verbal and spatial imagery tasks on eye fixations in driving. *J. Exp. Psychol. Appl., 6*(1), 31–43.

Schultheis, M. T., & Mourant, R. R. (2001). Virtual reality and driving: The road to better assessment of cognitively impaired populations. *Presence: Teleoperators and Virtual Environments, 10*(4), 436–444.

Schultheis, M. T., Garay, E., & DeLuca, J. (2001). The influence of cognitive impairment on driving performance in multiple sclerosis. *Neurology, 56*, 1089–1094.

Simone, L., Schultheis, M. T., Rebimbas, J., & Millis, S. R. (2006). Head Mounted Displays for Clinical Virtual Reality Applications: Pitfalls in understanding user behavior while using technology. *CyberPsychology and Behavior, 9*(5), 591–602.

Schultheis, M. T., Garay, E., Millis, S. R., & DeLuca, J. (2002). Motor vehicle violations and crashes in drivers with multiples sclerosis. *Arch. Phys. Med. Rehabil., 83*(8), 1175–1178.

Schultheis, M. T., Rebimbas, J., Mourant, R., & Millis, S. R. (2007). Examining the usability of a virtual reality driving simulator. *Assistive Technologies, 19*(1), 1–8.

Schultheis, M. T., Simone, L. K., Roseman, E., Nead, R., Rebimbas, J., & Mourant, R. (2006). Stopping behavior in a VR driving simulator: A new clinical measure for the assessment of driving? *IEEE Eng. Med. Biol. Sci.*, 4921–4924.

Summers, J. B. (2004 Feb.). Avoid lawsuits: Warn patients that medication may make them drowsy and not to drive. *J. Emerg. Nurs.*, *30*(1), 7–8.

Wingen, M., Bothmer, J., Langer, S., & Ramaekers, J. G. (2005 Apr.). Actual driving performance and psychomotor function in healthy subjects after acute and subchronic treatment with escitalopram, mirtazapine, and placebo: A crossover trial. *J. Clin. Psychiatr.*, *66*(4), 436–443.

Witman, A., Nieminen, T., & Summala, H. (1998). Driving experience and time-sharing during in-car tasks on roads of different width. *Ergonomics*, *41*, 358–372.

Woodward, L. J., Fergusson, D. M., & Horwood, L. J. (2000). Driving outcomes of young people with attentional difficulties in adolescence. *J. Am. Acad. Child. Adolesc. Psychiatr.*, *39*, 627–634.

van Zomeren, A. H., Brouwer, W. H., & Minderhoud, J. M. (1987). Acquired brain damage and driving: A review. *Arch. Phys. Med. Rehabil.*, *68*, 697–705.

Veeraraghavan, H., & Papaniklopoulos, N.P. (2001). Detecting driver fatigue through the use of advanced face monitoring techniques. Special report for the National Technical Information Service. Available at: http://www.ntis.gov.

Volna, J., & Sonka, K. (2006). Medical factors of falling asleep behind the wheel. *Prague Med. Rep.*, *107*(3), 290–296.

APPENDIX A

STATE REQUIREMENTS

		REQUIREMENTS					RENEWAL PROCEDURES		
	Visual acuity requirements in both eyes*	Absolute visual acuity minimum*	Corrective lenses allowed?	Additional visual requirements?		Bioptic telescopes allowed*	Length of license validation	Renewal options and conditions	Age-based renewal procedures?
				Minimum visual field	Color vision				
AL	20/40	20/60 in best eye restricted to daytime only	Yes	110 degrees in both eyes	Yes	Yes	4 years	In-person	No
AK	20/40	20/100 with report	Yes			Under certain conditions recommended by physician	5 years	Mail-in/ in-person	Yes
AZ	20/40	20/60 in best eye restricted to daytime only	Yes	70 degrees E, 35 degrees N		No	12 years	N/A	Yes
AR	20/50 with correction	20/40 in best eye	Yes	105 degrees in both eyes		20/50 through telescope and carrier, minimum field of vision 105 degrees	4 years	In-person, by mail only if out of state	None
CA	20/40	20/200 best corrected	Yes			Daylight driving only	5 years	In-person, mail-in	Yes
CO	20/40	20/70	Yes			Yes	10 years	In-person, if eligible mail-in every other cycle	Yes
CT	20/40	20/70 in best eye, allow 20/200 restricted	Yes	100 monocular/ 140 binocular		No	6 years	In-person	Yes
DE	20/40	20/50 restricted	Yes			Yes	5 years	In-person	None
DC	20/40 in best eye, 20/70 in better eye	20/40, 20/70 in better requires 140 E	Yes	130 degrees in both eyes		No	5 years	On-line w/ restrictions	Yes
FL	20/40 without correction	20/70	Yes	130 degrees horizontal		No	4–6 years depending on history	In-person 3rd cycle	Yes

			REPORTING					
Testing required at renewal?			Physician/medical reporting			Accept reporting from others?	Anonymity?	Immunity available?
Vision test	Written test	Road test	Required	Encouraged	None			
					x	Yes	No	Yes
x					Self-report	Yes	N/A	None
x		If recommended	x			Yes	Available	Available
x					x	Yes	N/A	None
At in-person renewal	At in-person renewal	If recommended	x			Yes	Available	Yes
At in-person renewal	Point accumulation results in suspension	No, unless condition has developed since last renewal			x	Yes	No	N/A
		For new applicants, expired more 2 years			x	Yes	Available	Yes
x			x			Yes	Available	Yes
x	x	Physical disabilities and senior citizens may be required			x	Yes	Available	None
In-person renewal	May be required based on history	May be required based on physical or mental impairments			x	Yes	Available	N/A

(Continued)

(Continued)

	Visual acuity requirements in both eyes*	Absolute visual acuity minimum*	Corrective lenses allowed?	Additional visual requirements?		Bioptic telescopes allowed*	Length of license validation	Renewal options and conditions	Age-based renewal procedures?
				Minimum visual field	Color vision				
	REQUIREMENTS						**RENEWAL PROCEDURES**		
GA	20/60	20/60 either eye with or without corrective lenses	Yes	140 degrees in both eyes		20/60 through telescope and carrier lens, 20/200 with restrictions	4 years	In-person	None
HI	20/40	20/40 in best eye	Yes	70 degrees in one eye		Permitted for use while driving	6 years	In-person/ mail-in	Yes
ID	20/40	20/40 in best eye	Yes			20/40 through lens, 20/60 through carrier	4 years	Mail-in	Yes
IL	20/40	20/40 in best eye	Yes	105 one eye/140 both eyes		Day light driving: carrier lenses 20/100 in better eye, 20/40 through bioptic telescope, 140 degrees binocular	4 years	In-person/ mail-in w/ restrictions	Yes
IN	20/40	20/40 in best eye	Yes	70 degrees in one eye, 120 degrees in both eyes		20/200 with some restrictions, if 20/40 can be achieved with telescope	4 years	In-person	Yes
IA	20/40	20/50 daylight only, 20/200 restriction	Yes	140 degrees both eyes		No	5 years	In-person	Yes
KS	20/40	20/60 in best eye maintain record 3 years	Yes	110 with both eyes/55 degrees monocular		Yes with eye doctor report	6 years	In-person	Yes
KY	20/40	20/200	Yes	120 degrees and 80 degrees in same eye		20/60 through telescope and 20/200 through carrier lens	4 years	In-person	None

		REPORTING			
Testing required at renewal?			Physician/medical reporting			Accept reporting from others?	Anonymity?	Immunity available?
Vision test	Written test	Road test	Required	Encouraged	None			
x			x			Yes	None	None
x		If necessary		x		Yes	N/A	None
x		If requested	x			Yes	None	None
x	8 years unless clean record	75+	x			Yes	Available	Yes
x	N/A	14+ points or 3 convictions in 12 mo. period			None, however require to report conditions to Board of Health within 60 days	Yes	N/A	None
x		If physical or mental conditions		x		Yes	None	Available
x	x	Visual Acuity of 20/60 or worse or at medical doctors request			x	Yes	None	N/A
			x			Yes	None	Yes

(*Continued*)

(Continued)

	Visual acuity requirements in both eyes*	Absolute visual acuity minimum*	Corrective lenses allowed?	Additional visual requirements?		Bioptic telescopes allowed*	Length of license validation	Renewal options and conditions	Age-based renewal procedures?
				Minimum visual field	Color vision				
LA	20/40	20/100 in better eye w/ restrictions	Yes			No	4 years	In-person/ mail-in/ Internet	Yes
ME	20/40	20/70 w/ restrictions	Yes	140 degrees both eyes, 110 degrees restricted		No	6 years	N/A	Yes
MD	20/40	20/100 w/ special permission	Yes	140 degrees continuous field of vision, 110 degrecs for restricted		20/70 through telescope and 20/100 carrier lens, restricted to daytime and requires outside mirrors	5 years	In-person	Yes
MA	20/40	20/70 best eye w/ restrictions	Yes	120 degrees	Yes	Vision at 120 degrees and acuity corrected 20/40 bioptic telescope and 20/100 carrier lens	5 years	In-person/ Internet	None
MI	20/40	20/70 in better eye with restriction	Yes	110–140 degrees in both eyes, less additional requirements		Road test required	4 years	Mail-in every other cycle, if free of convictions	No
MN	20/40	20/80 referred to driver evaluation unit	Yes	105 degrees		No	4 years	In-person	None
MS	20/40	20/70 w/ restriction	Yes	140 degrees in both eyes		Yes	4 years	In-person/ Internet	None
MO	20/40	20/160 w/ restriction	Yes	85 one eye w/ restrictions		Yes	6 years	In-person/ mail if out of state	Yes
MT	20/40	20/100 best eye w/ restriction	Yes			20/100 better carrier lens	4 years mail-in/8 years in-person	Mail-in / in-person	Yes

			REPORTING					
Testing required at renewal?			Physician/medical reporting			Accept reporting from others?	Anonymity?	Immunity available?
Vision test	Written test	Road test	Required	Encouraged	None			
x	Expired 1 year more	Expired 2 years or more		x		Yes	None, but can be requested by court order	Yes
At age 40, 52, 65 and every 4 years after			x			Yes	None	N/A
x			x			Yes	Available	N/A
x				x		Yes	None	N/A
x	x	Expired more than 4 years		x		Yes	None, but can be requested by court order	None
x	License expired more than 1 year	License expired more than 5 year		x		Yes	None, but can be requested by court order	Yes
x	N/A	N/A		x		Yes	N/A	No
x	if license has been expired for more than 6 months	if license has been expired for more than 6 months		x		Yes	Available	Yes
x	at discretion of examiner	at discretion of examiner		x		Yes	None, if requested state will disclose info	Yes

(*Continued*)

(Continued)

	Visual acuity require-ments in both eyes*	Absolute visual acuity minimum*	Corrective lenses allowed?	Additional visual requirements?		Bioptic telescopes allowed*	Length of license validation	Renewal options and conditions	Age-based renewal procedures?
				Minimum visual field	Color vision				
NE	20/40	20/70	Yes	140 degrees in both eyes		20/70 or better through telescope	5 years	In-person/ mail-in	None
NV	20/40	20/50 w/ restrictions	Yes	140 degrees binocular	None	20/40 through telescope, 20/120 through carrier lens, and 130 E visual field	4 years	Mail-in every other cycle	Yes
NH	20/40	20/70 w/ restrictions	Yes			Yes	5 years	N/A	Yes
NJ	20/50	20/50	Yes			20/50 through telescope	4 years	In-person	None
NM	20/40	20/40	Yes	120 degrees in external and 30 nasal field of one eye		No	4 or 8 years	N/A	Yes
NY	20/40	20/40	Yes	140 degrees E horizontal visual fields		20/80–20/100 corrected min 140 degrees E horizontal visual fields plus 20/40 through bioptic telescope lens	8 years	In-person/ mail-in	None
NC	20/40	20/100	Yes	60 degrees in one eye		No	5 years	In-person	Yes
ND	20/40	20/80 better eye if 20/100 in other eye	Yes	140 degrees in both eyes		20/130 through carrier lens, 20/40 through telescope, and full peripheral fields	4 years	In-person	None
OH	20/40	20/70 in best eye w/ restrictions	Yes	70 degrees in each eye	Yes	Yes	4 years	In-person/ mail if person out of state	None

Top spanning headers: REQUIREMENTS — RENEWAL PROCEDURES

	Testing required at renewal?			Physician/medical reporting			Accept reporting from others?	Anonymity?	Immunity available?
	Vision test	Written test	Road test	Required	Encouraged	None			
	x	License expired more than 1 year or suspended, revoked or cancelled	License expired more than 1 year or suspended, revoked or cancelled		x		Yes	None, unless driver appeals the denial or cancellation in court	No
	x	Unless license class has changed	Unless license class has changed	x			Yes	Available	Yes
	x				x		Yes	None	N/A
	Periodically	Recommended examiner	Recommended examiner	x			Yes	N/A	Yes
	x	May be required	May be required	x			Yes	None	Yes
	x				x		Yes	None	No
	x	x			x		Yes	None	Yes
	x				x		Yes	None	Yes
	x				x		Yes	None	No

(*Continued*)

(Continued)

	Visual acuity require-ments in both eyes*	Absolute visual acuity minimum*	Corrective lenses allowed?	Additional visual requirements?		Bioptic telescopes allowed*	Length of license validation	Renewal options and conditions	Age-based renewal procedures?
	REQUIREMENTS						**RENEWAL PROCEDURES**		
				Minimum visual field	Color vision				
OK	20/60	20/100 in best eye w/ restrictions	Yes	70 degrees in the horizontal meridian with both eyes together		No	4 years	In-person	None
OR	20/40	20/70 in best eye w/ restrictions	Yes	110 degrees in horizontal plane one or both eyes		Can be used only with carrier lens	8 years	Mail-in every other cycle	Yes
PA	20/40	20/70 w/ restrictions	Yes	120 degrees in both eyes		Permitted for driving, 20/100 or better with carrier lens only	4 years	Internet, mail, in-person	Yes
RI	20/40	20/40	Yes			N/A	5 years	Unknown	Yes
SC	20/40	20/40 in best eye	Yes	Total angle greater 140 degrees		Yes	5 years	In-person	None
SD	20/50	20/40 better eye	Yes			Driver must pass skill test	5 years	In-person	None
TN	20/40	20/60 with restrictions	Yes			20/200 better eye through carrier lens, 20/60 through telescope, visual field is 150 or greater, and magnification is no greater than 4x	5 years	In-person, mail, Internet	None
TX	20/40	20/70 in better eye w/ restrictions	Yes		New drivers	Client has 20/40 through telescope and passes road test	6 years	In-person, eligible by Internet, phone, mail	None
UT	20/40	20/100 in better eye w/ restrictions	Yes	90 degree binocular total with 45 both right and left		No	5 years	In-person, mail-in every other cycle w/ restrictions	Yes

| | Testing required at renewal? | | Physician/medical reporting (REPORTING) | | | Accept reporting from others? | Anonymity? | Immunity available? |
Vision test	Written test	Road test	Required	Encouraged	None			
				x		Yes	None	Yes
only after age 50			x			Yes	No	Yes
			x			Yes	Yes	Yes
x			x			Yes	N/A	Yes
x	Only if 5+ points	If appears to be needed		x		Yes	N/A	None
x				x		Yes	N/A	None
				x		Yes	N/A	Yes
In-person renewal				x		Yes	During administrative hearing be revealed	Yes
				x		Yes	None	Yes

(Continued)

(Continued)

	REQUIREMENTS						RENEWAL PROCEDURES		
				Additional visual requirements?					
	Visual acuity require-ments in both eyes*	Absolute visual acuity minimum*	Corrective lenses allowed?	Minimum visual field	Color vision	Bioptic telescopes allowed*	Length of license validation	Renewal options and conditions	Age-based renewal procedures?
VT	20/40	20/40 in better eye	Yes	Each eye 60 degrees, 60 degrees external and 60 degrees nasal for one eye only		Daytime driving only restriction and vehicle weight restriction (10,000lbs). Client must pass road test	2–4 years	Mail-in/ in-person	None
VA	20/40	20/40 in best eye	Yes	100 degrees monocular and binocular; 70 degrees monocular and binocular, restricted		20/200 through carrier lens and 20/70 through telescope. A test is required.	5 years	Mail-in, Internet, telephone, fax, extra teller	None
WA	20/40	20/40 in better eye	Yes	110 degrees horizontal	Yes	Yes	5 years	In-person	None
WV	20/40	20/40	Yes		Yes		5 years	In-person	None
WI	20/40	20/100 in better eye	Yes	70 degrees in better eye for regular unrestricted license		Used only in driving not to improve vision	8 years	In-person	None
WY	20/40	20/100 in better eye w/ restrictions	Yes	120 degrees binocular for new, renewal and professional drivers		20/100 or better through both carrier lenses, distance restriction for at least 1 year	4 years	In-person, mail-in every other	None

			REPORTING					
Testing required at renewal?			Physician/medical reporting			Accept reporting from others?	Anonymity?	Immunity available?
Vision test	Written test	Road test	Required	Encouraged	None			
				x		Yes	None	No
x	Two or more violations in 5 years			x		Yes	None	No
x	Pending on health screens	Pending on health screens		x		Yes	None	No
				x		Yes	None	No
x	Determined by DOT, vision specialist or physician	Determined by DOT, vision specialist or physician		x		Yes	None	Yes
x		Only warranted by physician		x		Yes	N/A	Yes

APPENDIX B

RESOURCES

BOOKS

Pellerito, J. M. (2006). Driver Rehabilitation and Community Mobility: Principles and Practice. St. Louis, Missouri: Elsevier Mosby Publishers.

Groeger, J. A. (2000). Understanding Driving: Applying Cognitive Psychology to a Complex Everyday Task. New York, NY: Psychology Press.

Stav, W. (2004). Driving Rehabilitation: A Guide for Assessment and Intervention. San Antonio, TX: Harcourt Assessment Inc.

Mann, W. (2006) Community Mobility: Driving and Transportation Alternatives for Older Drivers. Binghamton, NY: Haworth Press.

INTERNET: FREE DOWNLOADS

American Medical Association (AMA). (2003). Physician's Guide to Assessing and Counseling Older Drivers. http://www.ama-assn.org/ama/pub/category/10791.html

Canadian Medical Association (CMA). Determining Medical Fitness to Operate Motor Vehicles CMA Driver's Guide (Seventh edition). http://www.cma.ca/index.cfm/ci_id/18223/la_id/1.htm

Safety Mobility for Older People Notebook (1999). DOT Report # 808853 http://www.nhtsa.dot. gov/people/injury/olddrive/safe/safe-toc.htm

Model Driver Screening and Evaluation Program (2003). DOT Report # 809581 http://www.nhtsa. dot.gov/people/injury/olddrive/modeldriver/

INTERNET: WEB SITES

AAA FOUNDATION FOR TRAFFIC SAFETY

http://www.aaafoundation.org
This site covers a variety of topics for drivers as well as health professionals: Research information, online quizzes, and a good selection of brochures.

AMERICAN DRIVER AND TRAFFIC SAFETY
EDUCATION ASSOCIATION (ADTSEA)

http://adtsea.iup.edu/adtsea/default.htm
The ADTSEA is the professional association which represents traffic safety educators throughout the
United States and abroad.

AMERICAN OCCUPATIONAL THERAPY
ASSOCIATION: OLDER DRIVERS

http://www1.aota.org/olderdriver
A national professional association established that represents the interests and concerns of occupational therapy practitioners and students of occupational therapy and to improve the quality
of occupational therapy services. Driving rehabilitation is a subsection and area of specialty in
occupational therapy.

ASSOCIATION OF DRIVER EDUCATORS FOR
THE DISABLED

http://www.driver-ed.org
Leading national organization that supports professionals working in the field of driver education/
driver training and transportation equipment modifications for persons with disabilities through
education and information dissemination. Lots of helpful resources, including state-by-state
directory of certified driver specialist and disability and driving fact sheets.

ASSOCIATION FOR THE ADVANCEMENT OF
AUTOMOTIVE MEDICINE

http://www.carcrash.org/genlinfo.htm
An international multidisciplinary organization for crash injury control.

BRAIN INJURY ASSOCIATION OF AMERICA
(BIA)

http://www.biausa.org/publications/safedriving.htm
A national organization serving and representing individuals, families, and professionals who
affected by traumatic brain injury (TBI), offers information about brain injury and driving.

NATIONAL HIGHWAY TRAFFIC SAFETY
ADMINISTRATION

http://www.nhtsa.dot.gov
The "NHTSA" site includes information on their organization as well as vehicle and equipment
information, and traffic safety and occupant protection.

NATIONAL SAFETY COUNCIL

http://www.nsc.org/index.htm

A non-for-profit, charitable, international public service organization dedicated to educating and influencing people to prevent accidental injuries and deaths.

TRANSPORTATION RESEARCH BOARD (TRB)

http://www.trb.org

TRB is one of six major divisions of the National Research Council – a private, nonprofit institution that is the principal operating agency of the National Academies in providing services to the government, the public, and the scientific and engineering communities. TRB provides a leadership in transportation innovation and progress through research and information exchange, conducted within a setting that is objective, interdisciplinary, and multimodal.

TRANSPORTATION RESEARCH INFORMATION SERVICES (TRIS)

http://ntlsearch.bts.gov/tris/index.do

TRIS is a public-domain, web-based database. TRIS Online is published as a collaborative effort by the Transportation Research Board, part of the National Academies, and the National Transportation Library, part of Bureau of Transportation Statistics (BTS), Research and Innovative Technology Administration, (US Department of Transportation).

INDEX

Printed and bound by CPI Group (UK) Ltd, Croydon, CR0 4YY

03/10/2024

01040422-0004